Is It Me or My Hormones?

THE GOOD, THE BAD, AND THE UGLY ABOUT PMS, PERIMENOPAUSE, AND ALL THE CRAZY THINGS THAT OCCUR WITH HORMONE IMBALANCE

Marcelle Pick
MSN, OB/GYN NP

HAY HOUSE, INC.
Carlsbad, California • New York City
London • Sydney • Johannesburg
Vancouver • Hong Kong • New Delhi

Published and distributed in the United States by: Hay House, Inc.: www.hayhouse.com® • *Published and distributed in Australia by:* Hay House Australia Pty. Ltd.: www.hayhouse.com.au • *Published and distributed in the United Kingdom by:* Hay House UK, Ltd.: www.hayhouse.co.uk • *Published and distributed in the Republic of South Africa by:* Hay House SA (Pty), Ltd.: www.hayhouse.co.za • *Distributed in Canada by:* Raincoast: www.raincoast.com • *Published in India by:* Hay House Publishers India: www.hayhouse.co.in

Indexer: Jay Kreider, Index It Now
Cover design: Karla Baker • *Interior design:* Tricia Breidenthal

Charts on pages 11 and 12 and image on page 41 © Women to Women Personal Program, www.womentowomen.com

Cataloging-in-Publication Data is on file at the Library of Congress

Hardcover ISBN: 978-1-4019-4274-8
Digital ISBN: 978-1-4019-4275-5

16 15 14 13   4 3 2 1
1st edition, March 2013

Printed in the United States of America

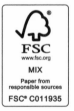

Praise for Marcelle Pick

"My day would begin with me feeling exhausted and having pains and aches throughout my body. Mood swings, nausea, irregular bowel discomfort, and a constant battle with inflammation and obesity accumulated over the years and left me drained and depressed. My recovery is due to the guidance of Marcelle Pick and her ability to teach the patient how to understand and support their individual needs and create health through nutrition, hormone balance, and spiritual awakening. This book's method has helped me lose more than 100 pounds, and I have more energy and joy than I can ever remember."

— Patricia Berube

"I have been a patient of Marcelle's for 15-plus years. Over the years, she has taught me considerably about health and opened my eyes to a healthy life. I was overweight for most of my adult life. With Marcelle's help, I lost 45 pounds. She never gave up on me. I was tipping the scales at 185 pounds and had tried many different diet plans. Her insights into my food cravings, hormone imbalance, sluggishness, and lack of energy were life altering. I now feel healthier than I have ever felt. Marcelle devised a supplement plan that has made a huge, positive difference in my life. I look forward to my yearly annual check-ins with Marcelle, as each time I visit with her, I know I will learn a tidbit more about becoming healthier. There's no other way to say it . . . Marcelle changed my life."

— Carol Hauser

"I have followed everything that Marcelle has advised me to do. I'm a woman on her journey."

— Barbara Lavigne

"I met with Marcelle Pick and she listened to me and worked out a program to get me feeling like me again. Since our first meeting, I am feeling like the old/new me again!"

— Mary Ann Benedict

"I have been a patient of Marcelle's for more than 20 years. The older I get, the more I appreciate her cutting-edge approach to women's health, her brilliant mind, and her commitment to my entire well-being. Over the years, as different issues have come up, Marcelle has always taken a multifaceted approach to finding the solutions. Marcelle knows me and what makes me tick. I could not ask for a better partnership in seeking optimal health than the one I have with Marcelle."

— Willo Wright

Is It Me or My Hormones?

ALSO BY MARCELLE PICK

The Core Balance Diet

Is It Me or My Adrenals?

To women around the world who
need to know the truth and to my children
who deserve to have a healthier world

CONTENTS

INTRODUCTION

It's Not You!

I'll never forget it.

I was 20 years old, having just graduated from college, home for the summer while preparing to take off for a long-awaited trip to Europe. My whole life lay ahead of me—and I wasn't even able to get motivated to renew my passport. Despite all the wonderful things I had to look forward to, I was miserable. I felt bloated and weighed down, physically and emotionally.

I remember sitting in my mother's car outside a pottery shop while she went inside. I was thinking about all the things I had to do: get my tickets, shop for new clothes, and call the close friend who would be traveling with me. This should have been an exciting time, so I couldn't understand why I felt so numb. Only a few days earlier, I had felt thrilled to be going off to explore this new chapter of my life. But now I was filled with despair. What in the world had happened to me?

Looking back on that bewildered 20-year-old, I wish I could tell her what I know now. I wish I could say to her, "I know you feel overwhelmed and confused. But there is a simple explanation. You're suffering from PMS, and the good news is that help is readily available."

MY HORMONAL JOURNEY

I struggled with hormonal issues throughout my 20s. Every month I wondered whether this one would be just difficult or a truly grueling ordeal. All too often, I felt like an alien had taken up residence inside me, bringing with it bloating, nausea, ravenous appetite, low energy, and terrible cramping. Usually I enjoyed life but not when this other entity paid its monthly visits.

When I became a nurse-practitioner, I discovered that I was far from alone. Many of my patients struggled with difficult PMS, painful periods, or challenging *perimenopause,* the transition into menopause that typically begins in the early or mid-40s and continues until menopause finally takes over. My patients were also dealing with endometriosis, fibroids, polycystic ovarian syndrome (PCOS), and premature ovarian failure (POF) and other fertility issues. Many women felt, as I did, that hormonal issues were playing far too big a role in their lives. We all longed for a straightforward solution.

As I continued my practice and began reading the literature in the field, I learned a great deal about healing both my patients and myself. To my amazement, I discovered that the right foods could keep our hormones in harmony, especially when aided by deep, restful sleep, energizing exercise, the right herbs and nutritional supplements, and, if necessary, some gentle bioidentical hormones. I found out the best ways to avoid environmental toxins that mimic the effects of estrogen and disrupt our hormonal balance. I learned how psychological stressors of all kinds—from everyday challenges to our family histories—affect our adrenal glands, and how our adrenals, in turn, are one of the keys to hormonal balance. (I even wrote a book on the topic: *Is It Me or My Adrenals?: Your Proven 30-Day Program for Overcoming Adrenal Fatigue and Feeling Fantastic Again.*) Having grown up with a father who was a psychologist and a mother who was a social worker, I was very much aware that psychological issues affect us, but I never fully appreciated their physical implications until I started working with women and their hormones. Most important, I learned how crucial it was to listen to our bodies—hormones and all—and to respect the messages they give us.

Eventually, my partner and I joined Christiane Northrup, M.D., and her partner to start a new practice. We kept the name I had first chosen, Women to Women, which I'm proud to say has become a national leader in the field of women's health. Drawing on the new perspectives we were all discovering together, Chris went on to write a landmark book, *Women's Bodies, Women's Wisdom,* which has helped transform the way women's health issues are regarded in this country and around the world.

Our groundbreaking work crystallized around the two key ideas I've mentioned: first, that our hormones are deeply affected by diet, lifestyle, and environmental influences—including the many toxins and pollutants in our food, air, and water—and second, that our understanding of the world and our place in it plays a hugely important role. A woman who rarely exercises and eats a diet high in sugar and the wrong kinds of fats is far more likely to have a challenging menstrual cycle than a woman who gets the right kind of exercise and eats a healthy balance of protein, carbs, healthy fats, and fiber. Similarly, a woman who has learned from her earliest childhood that her own needs must take a backseat to the needs of others is likely to experience an additional barrage of daily stress in her life—stress that has a powerful effect on her body chemistry, including her hormones.

The exciting news was that we could do a great deal to help these women, which became a lifelong passion for me. We could treat our patients' hormonal issues naturally, safely, and effectively, with near-miraculous effects on their overall health. It was amazing to see a woman whose month had been shadowed by mood swings, bloating, and cravings come into my office glowing, happy, and peaceful after just a few weeks of treatment. It was incredibly gratifying to hear our patients tell us, "Finally, I have periods without cramping" or "For the first time in a long time, I feel sexy and sensual again."

Many of the approaches we took were truly pioneering. We could see from our own experience the huge impact that nutrients had on physiology, even before there was widespread scientific evidence to back up that perception. Now, several decades later, such scientific support abounds. For example, the Harvard scientist Walter Willett, M.D., has shown clearly how deeply our bodies are affected by what we eat. Articles in the prestigious *New England Journal of Medicine* attest to the biochemical effects of stress upon our bodies and to the medical importance of relieving stress and/or transforming our responses to it. This cutting-edge work is wonderful validation for the medical approaches we developed and the exciting results we've achieved.

And so, finally, I began to make friends with my monthly cycle. I ate foods that were right for my body, slept a refreshing eight hours a night, and got moderate but vigorous exercise. I took herbs and nutritional supplements that were helpful for my particular biology. I explored the psychological issues that were adding unnecessary stress to my life and found new ways to get the support I needed. To my surprise, I discovered that my menstrual cycle was hormonally designed to include a creative, fruitful time in mid-cycle and then a quiet, peaceful, inward-turning time as my cycle reached its end. After balancing my hormones, I could finally enjoy the ebb and flow of my monthly cycle, appreciating its rhythms and shifts as women have done for generations.

My own experience brought home the huge role hormones play in how we feel. Now when I see women every day with concerns, questions, and frustrations about their hormones, I really get it. And when I hear women tell me that their hormonal struggles shape their lives—that they plan their months around mood swings and cramps, or that perimenopause is making them feel old before their time—I get that, too.

This suffering is simply not necessary. That's why I have written this book: to provide you with a simple, clear, accessible, 28-day program that can help you balance your hormones and make you feel like yourself again. We all deserve no less.

FUNCTIONAL MEDICINE: AN INTEGRATED APPROACH

This book comes out of a branch of medicine known as *functional medicine:* a holistic, integrated approach to the body and health. Whereas conventional medicine often tends to zero in on individual symptoms, make a diagnosis, and prescribe a treatment specifically targeted to that symptom or to the condition that immediately produced it, functional medicine casts a wider net. Our focus is less on symptoms and more on *systems* as we try to keep the entire matrix of the body in sight.

As a functional-medical practitioner looking at hormonal health, for example, I look at a patient's endocrine system (which produces all the body's hormones); neurotransmitters (biochemicals that affect mood, energy, and mental focus); the cardiovascular system; nutrition; lifestyle (exercise, sleep, and amount of stress); and psychological issues. As I consider information about all of those systems, I begin to piece together what interventions might be needed. Instead of looking "downstream" at the symptoms and how to treat them, I look "upstream" at the causes and how to transform them. After all, unless they've been in an accident of some kind, people do not go in a single day from perfect health to significant illness. Wellness and illness are a continuum we travel, with many factors affecting where along that continuum we fall.

One of the most important factors in health—perhaps the *most* important from a functional medicine point of view—is food. Accordingly, I view food as medicine, and one of my first concerns—as you'll see in this book—is to make sure that my patients are eating the foods that can make them well, and avoiding the foods that can make them sick. Sugar, refined carbohydrates, trans and hydrogenated fats, preservatives, and artificial ingredients can be particularly toxic and are often implicated in hormonal issues as well as in many other health concerns. My functional-medicine colleagues and I understand that we can literally use food to shift a patient's biochemistry, often with dramatic results.

In these pages, then, I'll talk you through the basic science of how hormones affect your body, mind, and emotions. I'll show you how to overcome hormonal symptoms, including weight gain, cravings, irritability, mood swings, and depression. I'll explain how rebalancing your hormones can help you lose weight and how it can do wonders for your skin, your hair, and your overall sense of vitality and well-being. I'll show you how to come to terms with the intense feelings associated with PMS and perimenopause so you can regain your emotional balance and learn the hidden significance of these psychological storms, as well as strategies for dealing with endometriosis, fibroids, and PCOS.

I will also help you understand the effects of the "body burden" of toxins and hormonal disrupters. This burden includes poor diet, lack of exercise, insufficient sleep, and psychological stress, but it also includes environmental toxins. These are pollutants that can be found in our food, water, and air. They are also present in many household cleaning products and such beauty care products as shampoo, moisturizer, and cosmetics. I'll show you how to relieve yourself of as much of that body burden as possible, which could make a huge difference in your hormonal health.

Finally, I'll help you restore your sensuality and sexuality so you can reclaim this important aspect of your identity and take pleasure in your body. Sex is such a wonderful part of life! Yet many of us face hormonal and psychological obstacles that keep us from fully enjoying our sexuality, our sensuality, and our intimate relationships. I'll show you how to rediscover your own vitality and sensuality and offer some suggestions for how to communicate more effectively with your partner.

Then, at the end of this book, you'll find a complete 28-day plan for rebalancing your hormones so you can once again enjoy the full experience of your life—every day of the month. I'll talk you through a hormone-healthy diet and lifestyle, with 28 days' worth of meal plans and recipes.

So welcome to your wonderful new world of hormonal health! No matter what your age, your weight, your medical condition, or your history, you *can* reclaim your body, your emotions, your energy, and your sex life. All you need is the right information and the willingness to begin. And how exciting is that?

Part I

UNDERSTANDING YOUR HORMONES

CHAPTER 1

Why Doesn't Anyone Believe Me?

Sasha was almost in tears. A restaurant manager in her mid-30s, she had been struggling for the past 15 years with severe PMS. During the week before her period she could always expect severe depression, food cravings, weight gain, and a general sense of feeling out of control.

"I've literally been to ten doctors," she told me. "Every one of them says, 'But your lab work is normal,' or 'You're just depressed,' or 'I can't find anything wrong with you.' But there must be something wrong with me! I'm a mess for one week every month—some months the symptoms last for two whole weeks. I'm hungry all the time. I have these weird cravings. I'm snapping at everybody. My mood swings are like something out of a bad TV show. The last doctor I saw wanted to put me on antidepressants, but I don't think I'm depressed. Well, okay, maybe right before my period, but the rest of the time I'm fine. I just don't get why no one can find out what's wrong!"

After graduating college, Celeste landed an internship with a public relations company. She was thrilled by this exciting opportunity—but worried about how her difficult periods would affect her work life. "My bleeding has always been heavy, but lately it's gotten just ridiculous—and my cramps are so painful I can't concentrate on anything else. I've been to a couple of gynecologists, but all my tests came back normal. One of them offered to put me on the pill, but I don't like the side effects. If I have to tough it out, I guess I can—but I really want to figure out what the problem is. I worry that something serious may be going on!"

Margarita was a financial analyst in her late 40s. For the past few years she had been gaining weight, struggling with thinning hair, and watching her skin start to sag. "My husband is a wonderful man," she told me, "and we used to have a great sex life. Lately, I can't even imagine having sex with him. Libido? What's that? And I've put on so much weight lately—what if I just keep getting heavier and heavier? Worst of all, sometimes I walk into a room to get something and I don't even remember what I came in for! But when I went to my doctor, she just told me that most of these changes are an inevitable part of getting older. Is this really what I have to look forward to?"

For all three of these women—Sasha, Celeste, and Margarita—imbalanced hormones were a very real problem. PMS, menstrual cramps, and perimenopause were playing havoc with their energy, their mood, their psyche, their appearance, their weight, their professions, and their sex lives. These women had gone to their health-care practitioners for help but they hadn't really gotten any. Instead, they'd been given the message that nothing was really wrong, that the problems they faced were just a normal part of a woman's life.

Thank goodness this isn't true. PMS, painful periods, and a difficult transition into perimenopause are often the result of a *hormonal imbalance*. When your hormones are balanced again, these problems can disappear. And balancing your hormones is surprisingly simple. You'll be amazed to discover you can do this through a combination of diet, herbs and supplements, lifestyle, and psychological support, in some cases complemented with some gentle bioidentical hormones. (You can find a step-by-step approach to balancing your hormones in the 28-day plan in the second part of this book.)

Now at this point, you may be wondering why, if these problems are so real and the solutions are so simple, your own health-care practitioner hasn't already given you this information. The answers to *that* question are not so simple. So let's take a closer look.

WHAT MOST HEALTH-CARE PRACTITIONERS MISS

You're gaining weight, feeling "off," and are frequently tired, irritable, and moody. During the week before your period, you may be subject to cravings, bloating, mood swings, weepiness, or anger. The week of your period, you get cramps and perhaps heavy bleeding. If you're in your 40s, you may be noticing more frequent problems with memory, focus, and mood, not to mention weight gain, sex drive, and what feels like the loss of your sensuality.

Your health-care practitioner may tell you that hormones fluctuate so frequently that it isn't worth testing them. If you are tested, you might be told that your estrogen and progesterone levels are in the normal range so there's nothing to worry about. Or your practitioner offers to prescribe the birth-control pill or some antidepressants.

You leave the office feeling frustrated and confused. Like Sasha, Celeste, and Margarita, you *know* that something's wrong. You want to feel vital, focused, energetic, at home in your own body. You want to feel sexy and sensual. And you don't understand why the person you trust to help you with your medical problems has just let you down.

So what's going on?

Unfortunately, all too often, the approach most conventional practitioners take misses the mark. Here are some reasons why.

1. Many practitioners look at too few hormones. When women struggle with PMS, painful periods, perimenopause, endometriosis, fibroids, or PCOS, most health-care practitioners look at the female sex hormones most immediately responsible for a woman's cycle: estrogen and progesterone. But these tell only part of the story—and often not even the most important part. If you are having problems with any of the conditions I just mentioned, three **other** hormones are almost certainly involved:

- **Cortisol and adrenaline:** stress hormones produced by the adrenal glands, which get involved every time you face a physical or emotional challenge

- **Insulin:** the hormone produced by the pancreas to help move blood sugar into your cells, which gets involved every time you eat a carbohydrate.

Without addressing these three hormones, your practitioner probably can't offer you an effective long-term solution. Yet most conventional practitioners don't even consider these hormones when treating "female complaints."

2. Many practitioners ignore the hormonal cascade. Your body contains more than 100 hormones and they all communicate with each other. If one hormone is off, it throws off another, and then another, creating a **hormonal cascade** of interrelated problems and symptoms.

A key hormonal cascade begins with cortisol, the stress hormone. When your adrenals produce either too much or too little cortisol, your other hormones feel it right away, including *thyroid* (which regulates metabolism), *leptin* (which regulates fullness), *ghrelin* (which regulates hunger), *insulin* (which regulates blood sugar), *serotonin* (a natural antidepressant that helps you feel calm and self-confident), *dopamine* (a "feel-good" hormone that helps you feel excited and energized), and many, many others. All of these hormones must work together to produce health, well-being, and vitality, so if your health-care practitioner isn't looking at the hormonal cascade, he or she isn't seeing the whole picture.

3. Many practitioners look at individual hormones rather than overall hormonal balance. Suppose you have "high-normal" estrogen and "low-normal" progesterone. Your practitioner is likely to tell you that you're in the normal range and that you have nothing to worry about. You don't understand how that can be because you are still struggling with PMS, painful periods, or the symptoms of perimenopause (memory problems, lack of focus, weight gain, loss of sex drive). What your practitioner has failed to look at is the balance **between** estrogen and progesterone. Perhaps your "high-normal" estrogen is too high for your "low-normal" progesterone. This lack of balance is known as **estrogen dominance** and it may be responsible for a lot of what you've been feeling.

4. Many practitioners look at symptoms rather than root causes. As a result, they might prescribe either the birth-control pill or an antidepressant, either of which might have some limited effectiveness in relieving your symptoms. Unfortunately, neither of these medications gets at the root of the problem. Your estrogen and progesterone likely went out of whack because of an imbalance in your cortisol, adrenaline, and insulin levels, which reflect diet, lifestyle, and the stresses in your life. Inflammation and toxicity might also be contributing factors. The pill and antidepressants are just Band-Aids that don't address the problem at the deepest, most helpful level.

When addressing symptoms and disorders, it's important to look at what's going on upstream, at the whole matrix of conditions that gives rise to hormonal imbalance and other health issues. This integrated approach allows us to look at antecedents and triggers as well as results.

5. Many practitioners underestimate the crucial impact of diet, lifestyle, and psychology on hormonal balance. After more than two and a half decades of practice, I'm still amazed at the near-miraculous impact of changing your diet. When a woman cuts out sugar, eats more protein and healthy fat, and takes the herbs and supplements her body needs, a myriad of health problems clear up almost immediately. Getting the right kind of exercise can also make a world of difference, as can seven to nine hours of restful, refreshing sleep per day. Another key issue is life stress—the challenges of family, relationships, work, and personal life. As a great deal of scientific research has shown, stress has a powerful effect on your body. Finding effective ways to modify stress is crucial to achieving hormonal balance and freeing yourself from many symptoms once and for all.

IT'S *NOT* JUST "IN YOUR HEAD"

You know your body and yourself better than anyone else does. If you think something isn't working properly, you are almost certainly correct. So let's look at three major types of hormonal imbalance that commonly plague women. I want you to see just how hormonal imbalance creates the symptoms you've been suffering from.

Premenstrual Syndrome (PMS)

Years ago, when I was first struggling with my own hormonal shifts, I had heard about PMS, but the condition and treatments for it were not well known at that time. These days, the term has become an almost humorous cliché for an out-of-control woman. That's unfortunate, but at least we are aware of the problem!

It turns out that PMS is very, very real. For example, if you feel ravenous one moment and bloated the next, that's not "all in your head." It's a function of dysregulated hormones, including *insulin,* the blood-sugar hormone; *ghrelin,* which regulates hunger; and *leptin,* which creates feelings of fullness.

Similarly, the cravings you experience are not just based on feelings, and the weight gain that frustrates you is not a matter of willpower. These conditions have a biological basis. And if your weight fluctuates and you retain fluids, that's because of disrupted production of *thyroid hormone,* as well as the effects on your kidneys of excessive stress hormones, including *cortisol, adrenaline,* and *noradrenaline.*

Finally, if your mood, energy, focus, and concentration swerve all over the place, that's because your hormones affect your neurotransmitters, the biochemicals that allow for communication within the nervous system. If you crave sugar, sweets, and starches, that's partly because of the ways hormones affect your brain's response to another neurotransmitter called *serotonin.* Anxiety, depression, and mood swings can likewise result from imbalanced levels of stress hormones, serotonin, and other neurotransmitters, including *dopamine.*

One way that PMS can work is to strip away your defense mechanisms, leaving you far more vulnerable than usual to emotions that otherwise lie well below the surface. In that sense, you might think of PMS as your wake-up system, intensifying your emotions to help you confront something you otherwise might have missed. PMS might even offer some insights and messages about your life that you may want to listen to. To hear those messages clearly, however, it helps to ease your symptoms—both physical and emotional—with improved nutrition, sleep, and exercise, as well as with supplements (and, in some cases, bioidentical hormones; more about that in Chapter 4). Then, when emotions come up, you'll have the physical and emotional resources to evaluate the situation and take action.

The stakes are especially high because your current experience with PMS predicts your likely experience with perimenopause and menopause down the road. An easy cycle now probably means an easy transition later. Hormonal challenges now often predict problems later. The good news is that the help you give your hormones today through diet, lifestyle, and psychological support can also be a real game changer down the road.

Painful Periods

Anyone who has suffered through even a few hours of intense cramping knows how bad the pain can be. Even if you've experienced only mild discomfort during your period, you might still find yourself dividing up the month into "before," "during," and "after." When your estrogen and progesterone are out of balance, you might experience cramping, bloating, breast tenderness, mood swings, and a host of other symptoms.

What throws your estrogen and progesterone out of balance? A wide variety of factors might be involved, including diet, lack of exercise, environmental toxins, and the current or past use of birth-control pills. Imbalance might also result from excessive stress hormones flooding your body, perhaps in response to an overscheduled life, the press of too many deadlines, or an unrelenting set of emotional demands from the people around you.

Once again, restoring balance to the estrogen-progesterone relationship is relatively easy. As we'll see, diet, lifestyle, supplements, and, occasionally, bioidentical hormones can make a world of difference. So can looking at the sources of stress in your life and figuring out new ways to minimize, cope with, or even eliminate them.

Painful periods may also be the result of endometriosis. For more on endometriosis, see page 21.

Perimenopause

The transition from fertility to menopause is known as perimenopause—a gradual hormonal shift that usually begins in the late 30s or early 40s and extends into menopause. Perimenopause might be a relatively smooth transition as hormone levels adjust in preparation for the time when the menstrual cycle will end and a new era of life will begin. Or it might be a mini-preview of the worst aspects of menopause, including brain fog, mood swings, decreased libido, weight gain, night sweats, loss of vitality, and even hot flashes.

By paying attention to hormonal balance, you can sail through your 40s and 50s as an energetic, sensuous, and sexually alive woman, reaping the benefits of age and experience while enjoying the vitality of youth. Again, this is a perspective that many conventional practitioners miss. They offer perimenopausal women antidepressants, the birth-control pill, or pharmaceutical hormones made from horse urine, failing to see the big picture and ignoring the importance of diet, lifestyle, and modifying stress.

I successfully treat countless women who couldn't get help elsewhere. I work with them to change their diets and their lifestyles, offering them topical progesterone (a skin cream that contains small amounts of progesterone) and prescribing such nutritional supplements as evening primrose oil, essential fatty acids, and a high-quality multivitamin. I also use such herbs as black cohosh, red clover, wild yam, and chasteberry. I've witnessed firsthand how these natural treatments have given women back their lives as their painful symptoms disappear and the health problems that have plagued them since their teens resolve. This is the kind of help I'd like to offer you, too.

Hormones: Not Just a Women's Problem

Although this book is not dedicated to men, I want to take a moment to mention that men can have serious hormonal issues as well. Environmental toxins known as *xenoestrogens* imitate the effects of estrogen in the body and may increase men's estrogen levels while decreasing their testosterone levels. Aging can also contribute to this imbalance. Testosterone is especially important for muscle building, clear thinking, and cardiovascular protection, while increased estrogen leads to decreased sexual function, loss of motivation, and weight gain, often in the form of a pot belly. The beauty of all this is that men as well as women can benefit from a hormone-balancing 28-day plan, which contributes to weight loss, improved sexual function, increased energy and motivation, and improved cardiovascular health. So feel free to share this book with the men in your life!

HORMONES: YOUR BODY'S MESSENGER SYSTEM

The word *hormone* comes from the Greek word meaning "messenger." You can think of your body's many hormones as part of an elaborate messenger system, dashing through your bloodstream to share information, give instructions, and coordinate functions among your organs and nervous system. Unfortunately, when your hormones are out of balance, their messages can be muted, misunderstood, short-circuited, or garbled. If you're eating a diet high in sugar or low in the right kinds of fats, for example, you're not giving your hormones the support they need to carry clear, helpful messages. On the other hand, when you're eating a hormone-friendly diet, these messengers can be better understood by the rest of your body.

This is crucial because your hormones affect *everything:* your mood, your mental focus, your energy, your sex drive; your hair, your skin, your breasts, your vagina; your bones, your muscles, your heart, your brain . . . There really isn't any part of your mind, body, or spirit that isn't somehow affected by your hormones.

Major Female Endocrine Glands and Their Hormones
(a partial list)

Gland/organ	Hormone(s) released
Hypothalamus	• thyrotropin-releasing hormone • release inhibiting hormones
Pituitary	• thyrotropin/thyroid-stimulating hormone (TSH) • adrenocorticotropic hormone (ACTH) • luteinizing hormone (LH) • follicle-stimulating hormone (FSH) • growth hormone (GH) • prolactin • melanocyte-stimulating hormone (MSH) • oxytocin • antidiuretic hormone (ADH, or vasopressin)
Pineal	• melatonin
Thyroid and parathyroid	• thyroxine (T4) • triiodothyronine (T3) • calcitonin (CT) • parathyroid hormone (PH)
Thymus	• thymosin • thymopoietin • serum thymic factor
Adrenals	• epinephrine • norepinephrine • testosterone • estrogen • dehydroepiandrosterone (DHEA) • aldosterone • cortisol • corticosterone
Pancreas (islets of Langerhans)	• insulin • glucagon • somatostatin (also secreted elsewhere)
Ovaries	• estrone • estradiol • estriol • progesterone • testosterone
Placenta	• human chorionic gonadotropin (hCG)
Breasts	• estrogen

The Diffuse Endocrine System (other organs and tissues that secrete hormones)	
Tissue/organ	**Hormone(s) released**
Adipose tissue (fat) (Note that with development of truncal obesity, adipose tissue begins to function as a major player in the endocrine system.)	• leptin • adiponectin • resistin • plasminogen activating inhibitor–1 (PAI–1) • estrogen • and others
Skin	• vitamin D3 (cholecalciferol)
Stomach and small intestine	• gastrin • secretin • cholecystokinin • ghrelin • motilin
Liver	• 25–hydroxycholecalciferol
Kidneys	• erythropoietin (EPO) • 1,25-dihydroxycholecalciferol • rennin
Heart	• atrial naturetic hormone

Just as your hormones affect everything, they are also affected *by* everything. What you eat, drink, breathe, and put on your skin all affect your hormones. So do what you think, how you feel, how you grew up, and what you expect might happen next. That's why it's so crucial to take an integrated approach to your hormones. If you don't keep the whole picture in mind, you're likely to miss something really important.

Your hormones also profoundly affect one another, which is why balance is so important. Your hormones act like a symphony, in which every instrument needs to be playing just the right notes at just the right volume and the right tempo. No one element should be too loud or too soft, too slow or too fast. Only when every instrument plays its proper part can the orchestra achieve a beautiful, harmonious balance.

Your sex hormones are like the string section: they play an essential role in your anatomy, with profound effects on your body, mind, and emotions. Each hormone has multiple effects, both when it is in balance and when its levels are off. Here is a brief look at the four key sex hormones and a partial list of the ways they influence our health and well-being.

The Major Sex Hormones and Their Key Effects
Effects of Estrogen
Helps form neurotransmitters; improves mood; decreases depression, anxiety, irritability, and sensitivity to pain
Supports memory
Supports libido
Regulates blood pressure, increases blood flow, helps keep arteries elastic; reduces risk of heart disease by 40 to 50 percent
Reduces inflammation
Increases insulin sensitivity
Increases metabolism
Decreases LDL ("bad" cholesterol)
Maintains bone density
Maintains muscle
Decreases wrinkles and supports collagen, which keeps skin looking youthful
Protects against macular degeneration, an age-related eye disorder
Symptoms of Estrogen Deficiency
Difficulty losing weight despite diet and exercise
Increased insulin resistance
Vaginal dryness
Vulvodynia (vaginal pain)
Decrease in sexual interest and sexual function
Decrease in breast size
Polycystic ovarian syndrome
Low energy
Chronic fatigue syndrome
Memory problems
Anxiety
Depression

Bladder problems: more frequent infections, stress incontinence, and urge incontinence
Food cravings
Effects of Progesterone
Balances estrogen
Helps build bone
Supports healthy sleep
Helps prevent anxiety, irritability, and mood swings
Promotes healthy bladder function
Decreases palpitations
Relaxes the smooth muscle in the gut, allowing food to be digested more efficiently
Symptoms of Progesterone Deficiency
Weight gain
Heavy periods that last longer than seven days
Midcycle spotting
Irritability
Anger prior to menses
Menstrual migraines
Mood swings
Depression
Anxiety
Insomnia
Decreased libido
Decreased HDL ("good" cholesterol)
Pain and inflammation
Effects of Testosterone
Decreases extra body fat

Increases muscle mass and strength
Promotes well-being
Supports sexual interest
Supports neurotransmitters to combat depression
Helps maintain memory
Helps prevent bone deterioration
Symptoms of Testosterone Deficiency
Weight gain
Decline in muscle tone and increased muscle wasting despite adequate consumption of calories and protein
Decreased sex drive
Anxiety
Hypersensitivity or hyperemotional states
Mild depression
Fatigue
Less dreaming
Decreased HDL ("good" cholesterol)
Dry, thin, and less elastic skin
Dry, thinning hair
Saggy cheeks
Loss of pubic hair
Low self-esteem
Effects of DHEA
Healthy weight loss
Increased lean body mass
Lower cholesterol
More resources to deal with stress
Increased brain function

Reduced insulin resistance and more even blood sugar levels
Improved immune function and fewer allergic reactions
Increased sense of well-being
Improved body repair and maintenance
Symptoms of DHEA Deficiency
Weight gain
"Road rage," irritability, and difficulty dealing with stress
Decreased energy
Decreased muscle strength
Joint soreness
Increased risk of infection

HORMONE DISRUPTION IS REAL . . . BUT NOT INEVITABLE!

Now that we've established that hormone imbalances are real, we need to remind ourselves that they are not an inevitable part of being a woman. PMS, painful periods (medically known as *dysmenorrhea*), and challenging perimenopause are what goes wrong when there is a problem—which means that they disappear when the problem is resolved. Such disorders as endometriosis, fibroids, and polycystic ovarian syndrome are also signs of hormonal imbalance and may also clear up when you are able to rebalance your hormones. And if your periods have stopped *(amenorrhea)* or are extremely irregular, hormonal balance can go a long way toward helping you achieve more regularity and less discomfort. Finding and maintaining hormonal balance is within every woman's reach.

Before you can resolve your hormonal issues, however, you first need to understand the role they're playing in your life. Following are two questionnaires on the topic, one for PMS and one for perimenopause. Take some time to answer the questions to evaluate your hormonal health.

ARE YOUR HORMONES OUT OF BALANCE? THESE TWO QUESTIONNAIRES CAN HELP PROVIDE THE ANSWER

Take the following questionnaires to determine your degree of difficulty with PMS and perimenopause.

PMS

To qualify as PMS-related, the following symptoms must appear only one or two weeks before your period, beginning either during ovulation or during the week before your period and ending at menses or within one and three days after your period begins.

Rate the symptoms below according to the following system:

0 = no trouble / 1 = mild / 2 = moderate / 3 = severe / 4 = extreme

Abdominal cramping =

Agitation =

Anger =

Anxiety =

Avoiding social activities =

Backache =

Binge eating/cravings/food or alcohol overuse =

Bloating =

Breast tenderness or pain =

Constipation =

Decreased desire to talk with anyone =

Decreased libido =

Decreased work performance =

Depression =

Difficulty with relationships =

Fatigue/tiredness =

Fluid retention =

Headache =

Hopelessness =

Insomnia =

Mood swings =

Overreaction/irritability =
Poor judgment =
Poor self-esteem =
Sadness =
Tearfulness =
Tension =
Weight gain =

Scoring

0–4: Congratulations! You have almost no difficulties with PMS, indicating that your hormones are well balanced and your transition into perimenopause is likely to be smooth.

5–28: You have mild PMS, suggesting some difficulties with hormonal balance. Addressing this issue now will help you during your menstrual cycle and will make it more likely for you to have a gentle transition into perimenopause.

29–56: You are struggling with moderate PMS, compromising your ability to function optimally and to enjoy life for one or two weeks every month. Reading and working through this book should help end your symptoms.

57–84: Your PMS is so severe that it significantly affects the quality of your life. Following the suggestions in this book can make an immediate difference in helping you overcome your symptoms, setting you up for a much easier transition into perimenopause.

85–112: You are suffering from extreme PMS, to the point where your life may be organized around your symptoms. Your pain is real—but it does not need to continue. Following the 28-day program in Part II of this book can bring you relief, now and throughout perimenopause.

Perimenopause/Hormonal Imbalance

Unlike PMS-related symptoms, perimenopausal symptoms last the whole month long, although you may notice fluctuations based on your cycle or other factors.

Rate the symptoms below according to the following system:

0 = no trouble / 1 = mild / 2 = moderate / 3 = severe / 4 = extreme

Bloating =

Cravings =

Decreased libido =

Feeling anxious/heart palpitations/anxiety attacks =

Feeling asexual or completely unsensuous =

Feeling sad/moody/overwhelmed =

Frequent urination/incontinence when you laugh, cough, exercise, or jump =

Hot flashes/night sweats =

Irregular menses =

Irritability =

Loss of focus/foggy thinking =

Memory loss =

Osteoporosis/osteopenia =

Painful intercourse =

Skin changes/more wrinkling =

Skin feeling crawly =

Sleep difficulty/insomnia =

Sore breasts =

Stiff or achy joints =

Thinning hair =

Urinary tract infections =

Vaginal dryness =

Vaginal itching =

Weight gain =

Scoring

0–2: Congratulations! You have almost no difficulties with perimenopause because your hormones are well balanced.

3–23: You are struggling with mild hormonal imbalance, which is likely to get worse as your journey through perimenopause continues. Use the information in this book to correct the imbalance and restore yourself to full hormonal health.

24–46: You are suffering from moderate hormonal imbalance, which is affecting your quality of life. The pages ahead can help you restore balance to your hormones, eliminate your symptoms, and improve your daily life.

47–69: Your hormonal imbalance is so significant that it is seriously compromising your ability to function and enjoy your life. Restoring hormonal balance will improve your mood and replenish your energy.

70–96: You are suffering from extreme hormonal imbalance, which has become so serious that you scarcely remember what it was like to feel "normal." You frequently ask yourself, "Is it me or my hormones?" A great deal of your distress *is* caused by your hormones—and you can alleviate your discomfort significantly by following the 28-day program in the second part of this book.

DON'T KILL THE MESSENGER!

Your body may be sending you lots of uncomfortable messages, but the best way to begin to ease your discomfort is to listen to those signals. They're giving you important information about the way your life is changing, how you truly feel, and what your body needs. Are you eating too much sugar and not enough fiber? Your hormones will let you know. Are you short on sleep and long on stress? Your hormones will be the first to tell you. Are you too worried about pleasing your mother, your boss, your boyfriend, or your kids, and not worried enough about pleasing yourself? Your hormones will often give you information that even your best friends won't!

If we could just take time to listen to the ebb and flow of our hormones, we would be so much better off! *I'm so tired:* instead of reaching for the caffeine or the energy drink, when we hear that voice we should take a nap. *I'm so irritable:* again, maybe we should ask ourselves *why?* What is so annoying? What is irritating us so badly? *That's driving me crazy!!!:* what's going on for us when the irritability becomes full-blown rage? How much of our emotional response is based on what's happening now, as opposed to rehashing old battles with parents or siblings? Our hormones can help alert us to these issues and open us up to new insights.

All too often, we listen to other people instead of ourselves. We let ourselves be talked out of our emotions, our insights, and our experience. We put other people's needs first, and maybe we adopt—or try to adopt—other people's opinions as well. We try to be the person someone else wants us to be, or we try to fit some ideal we were taught long ago.

Our bodies—modulated by our hormones—will help remind us of how we really feel, what we really need, and who we really are.

Conditions Resulting from Hormonal Imbalance and/or Poor Estrogen Metabolism

Endometriosis. Every month, the uterus produces an *endometrium,* a thick lining intended to support a fertilized egg during pregnancy. If the egg is not fertilized and the woman doesn't become pregnant, the uterus is supposed to slough off the lining: this is the bleeding that occurs during your period. Endometriosis occurs when endometrial cells implant and grow outside the uterus. These endometrial implants can contribute to fertility issues and increased menstrual pain. Some 3 to 10 percent of all women have endometriosis, while 9 to 50 percent of infertility is caused by this condition. A significant body of evidence associates endometriosis and high levels of *dioxins,* a type of environmental toxin.

Fibroids are noncancerous tumors that grow from the muscle layers of the uterus, where they can produce excessive bleeding during the menstrual cycle. Some 20 percent of all U.S. women will develop fibroids at some point in their lives. Research has shown that women with fibroids tend to have an imbalance between estrogen levels that are too high and progesterone levels that are too low. Overweight or obese women have a higher risk of developing fibroids than women of a healthy weight.

Polycystic ovarian syndrome (PCOS). This very common female endocrine (hormone) disorder is characterized by irregular periods, lack of periods (amenorrhea), infertility, acne, hirsutism (growth of excess hair on the face and body), obesity, and high cholesterol. Compelling research links PCOS with insulin resistance. The condition is named for the benign ovarian cysts that appear in association with it, but the key features of the syndrome concern hormone levels, especially those of insulin, testosterone, estrogen, and progesterone.

I want to support you in trusting your feelings, your perceptions, and yourself. If your body is giving you a message, I want to help you listen. But this becomes much easier when you give your hormones the nourishment they need: lean proteins, high-fiber and low-glycemic carbs, the right types of healthy fats, a wide assortment of vitamins and minerals, and some specific nutrients such as the *sulfurofane* found in cruciferous vegetables—broccoli, cauliflower, cabbage, and Brussels sprouts. (You'll hear more about how to nourish your hormones in Chapter 4.)

Provide your hormones with the deep, restful sleep they require and try to protect them from the environmental toxins that stress your body (taxing your adrenals and generating the often disruptive hormone cortisol) and mimic or block estrogen (potentially disrupting your estrogen-progesterone balance). (You'll learn more about environmental toxins in Chapter 6.)

Support your hormonal balance by practicing the de-stressing activities that restore your spiritual and mental health: yoga, meditation, and any other spiritual practices that appeal to you. Perhaps most important, learn what stresses you out and why, going back into your family history to discover which stresses have more to do with your past than your present.

You can't enjoy your life when you're plagued by hormonally induced mood swings, cravings, heavy bleeding, or fatigue. You can't enjoy your sex life if unbalanced hormones are playing havoc with your libido, your mood, and the condition of your vagina. And you can't move forward with your life if your hormones are keeping you from thinking clearly, responding rationally, or staying focused.

My goal is to help you balance your hormones so that you can get on with the business of living. If you have only mild symptoms, just a few tweaks to diet and lifestyle may be enough. More significant symptoms might call for bigger changes—but they will also produce bigger results. And of course, whatever your current state, following through on suggestions that include diet, lifestyle, herbs, supplements, and stress reduction will bring you enormous rewards in terms of weight loss, appearance, vitality, sexuality, and sensuality.

So let's get started! Our next step is to move on to Chapter 2 so that we can fully understand the key players in your hormonal symphony.

CHAPTER 2

Your Hormonal Symphony

Lara was a nurse in her mid-30s who worked the emergency room's night shift. Hoping to be pregnant soon, she'd been putting in overtime so that she and her husband would have some extra money when the baby came. A cheerful, sociable person, Lara enjoyed her work, but on her days off she tended to skimp on sleep so she'd have more waking hours to spend with her friends and her husband. When she was working, Lara often went for hours without eating and then had a big meal at the end of her shift, usually something starchy and filling like pasta, pancakes, or French toast.

After several months of trying, Lara still hadn't gotten pregnant and came to me for help. When I asked her about her monthly cycle, she told me she'd been having somewhat irregular periods and a few mild but persistent PMS symptoms: some weepiness and depression for a few days before her period, occasional cravings for sweets, and some minor but noticeable bloating.

"Obviously I'm super-hormonal, right?" Lara said in her typical blunt, cheerful fashion. "That explains both the PMS and the trouble getting pregnant. So I'm guessing you want to do something to get my female hormones back into shape! Estrogen, progesterone—those are the hormones to fix, right?"

"Well, yes," I replied, "those are important. Both your PMS and your fertility issues may be related to imbalanced estrogen and progesterone, but of course many other factors might be involved."

Lara nodded. "Okay, so let's at least take care of the sex hormones!"

"Those may be the *immediate* cause," I reiterated, "but they probably aren't the *ultimate* cause. To get to the root of the problem there are some other hormones we have to look at. For example, your job is very stressful and you're working extra hours. Your body can handle stress in bursts, but you've been dealing with a lot for a long time, basically without a break. So I'm wondering if your *stress hormones—cortisol* and *adrenaline*—may be either too high or too low a lot of the time."

"I wouldn't be surprised," Lara said, shrugging. "But I'm not sure what difference that would make."

"When your estrogen and progesterone are out of balance, it's often because your stress hormones went out of balance first," I explained. "Stress hormones are incredibly powerful and they affect just about every bodily function—including your menstrual cycle. They may be a contributing factor keeping you from getting pregnant."

Lara looked at me in surprise.

"*Insulin* is another key hormone to look at," I told her. "Insulin regulates blood sugar. When you skip meals, that causes your blood sugar to drop. When you eat something sweet or starchy, especially on an empty stomach, that causes your blood sugar to spike. That crash-and-spike cycle is throwing your insulin out of balance."

"I didn't think I had to worry about insulin," Lara said. "I know I'm not diabetic."

"I know," I said, "but blood sugar and insulin imbalances affect us all. And imbalanced insulin also contributes to PMS symptoms. Plus, insulin imbalance is yet another type of stress on your system—which means it creates more stress hormones."

"Wow," Lara said. "It's a vicious cycle."

"Exactly," I said. "So between your stress hormones and your insulin, there are a lot of factors throwing your estrogen and progesterone out of balance. If we can rebalance your stress hormones and your insulin, a lot of your estrogen-progesterone issues will probably clear up by themselves."

"Sounds good," said Lara, cheerful again. "So where do we start?"

I explained to Lara the basics of the 28-day plan in the second part of this book. Diet, herbs and supplements, exercise, sleep, and psychological support go a long way toward balancing both stress hormones and insulin. And when those master hormones are in good balance, the rest of your hormones are far more likely to fall in line, too.

Lara embraced my 28-day plan with her usual enthusiasm, and the following month she saw an immediate improvement in her PMS symptoms. She continued to eat, sleep, and exercise in a hormone-friendly way, and she also took time to explore some personal issues that were adding extra stress to her life. She built in more quiet time for herself and added massage to her weekly schedule.

Within three months, Lara's periods were completely regular and she was symptom free. And three months after that, she was pregnant. Balancing her hormones through diet, lifestyle, and psychological support had made all the difference.

You can modify stress by . . .

- Getting seven to nine hours of restful sleep each night

- Doing moderate "bursting" exercise 20 minutes a day, four days a week (see page 63 for more detail)

- Avoiding as far as possible the environmental toxins that stress your system, particularly those that mimic the effects of estrogen (see Chapter 6)

- Reaching out to loved ones, friends, and community

- Being outdoors

- Getting a pet or spending time with animals

- De-stressing with such activities as massage, yoga, meditation, "me time," spiritual activities, time in nature, journaling, and other ways of reconnecting to yourself

- Engaging in blissful activities that give you pleasure, such as dancing, singing, reading, hiking, playing with children, group or community activities, or sex

- Treating yourself with as much compassion as you show others

- Developing your relationship to spirituality

- Exploring sources of stress and ways to cope differently, including journaling, a support group, therapy, and various mind-body modalities, such as art or dance therapy, Emotional Freedom Technique, Byron Katie's "The Work," and the Quadrinity Process (see Appendix D for further suggestions)

MEET YOUR HORMONAL ORCHESTRA

As we saw in Chapter 1, your hormones work together in an intricate dynamic not unlike that of a symphony orchestra. In an orchestra, some sections are more dominant than others at various times but the overall effect must be balanced and harmonious. If the string section goes astray, for example, it will quickly throw the whole orchestra off.

As Lara discovered, if your stress hormones or your insulin go out of balance, that's likely to cause significant problems elsewhere in your system, including your sex hormones: estrogen, progesterone, testosterone, and DHEA. These hormones regulate fertility, your menstrual cycle, and your transition into perimenopause, as well as your sex drive and your overall sense of sensuality. They also contribute to the development of muscle and many other important functions. Clearly, your sex hormones are a crucial part of any difficulties you might be having with PMS, painful periods, the transition into perimenopause, endometriosis, fibroids, and PCOS, not to mention any loss of interest in sex or feelings of being unsexy or unsensual. But without balancing your stress hormones and your insulin, you will find it nearly impossible to balance your sex hormones.

Because your hormones are a symphony, we can't just add one hormone at a time as if it weren't going to affect all the other players. Every hormonal prescription that we make will potentially have a significant ripple effect. To be successful in our treatment, we always need to look at the whole.

HORMONES, HORMONES EVERYWHERE

A wonderful book by neuroscientist Candace Pert called *Molecules of Emotion* makes it clear that we have receptors for neurotransmitters not just in the brain but everywhere in the body. This means that when your hormones go out of balance, your entire body feels the strain. Your mood, sexual energy, and overall energy are definitely affected, and I have even had patients tell me, "My eyes feel funny" or "My taste buds are off." On the other hand, when your hormonal symphony is playing in tune, your whole body feels the benefits.

THE IMPORTANCE OF HEALTHY FATS

Here's something most of my patients are very surprised to learn: the substance in the body from which our sex hormones are made is *cholesterol*. That's right. Cholesterol. Over the past few decades, we've learned to take a more nuanced approach to this villain of health care. We've all heard about the dangers of high cholesterol but it can also be a problem when it's too low. This is because without adequate cholesterol, the body can't make sufficient amounts of hormones. Similarly, without essential fatty acids (found in fish oil, flax oil, olive oil, nuts, and seeds) your body can't produce the hormones it needs.

Many of us have enough fat content in our diets to make healthy levels of hormones, but for some people on low-fat diets and/or on cholesterol-lowering statin medications, low cholesterol can be a problem. If your overall cholesterol is less than 150 and your LDL is less than 60, you might want to check with a nutritionist or a functional medicine practitioner to make sure you're not compromising your body's ability to make hormones.

CORTISOL AND ADRENALINE: THE MAJOR STRESS HORMONES

Stress hormones are so important to our overall health and well-being that there are many books on the subject, including my own: *Is It Me or My Adrenals?: Your Proven 30-Day Plan for Overcoming Adrenal Fatigue and Feeling Fantastic Again*. The term "stress" includes both physical stressors (such as lack of sleep, a recent or chronic illness, or over-work) and emotional stressors (such as deadline pressure, anxiety about a relationship, feeling upset about being yelled at, or the frustration of being cut off in traffic).

The stress response is regulated by a pair of glands known as the *adrenals*. When we are confronted with stress of any kind, our adrenals mobilize our bodies for the so-called "fight or flight" response, in which we prepare to do battle or flee. Among other hormones, the adrenals release adrenaline and cortisol into the bloodstream. The adrenaline prompts our heart rate to soar, our muscles to tense, and our mind to race. The cortisol increases glucose in the bloodstream and curbs nonessential functions such as digestion and reproduction. After all, if our lives are at risk—if we have to fight or flee—this isn't the time for food or sex!

Some Key Players in Your Hormonal Symphony

Here's a bird's-eye view of some key hormones and some of their most important functions. Every hormone performs many roles within your body, but for the purposes of this book, I'm providing you with a simplified summary of the key information to focus on:

- *Cortisol:* regulates stress

- *Adrenaline:* regulates stress

- *Thryoid:* regulates metabolism

- *Insulin:* regulates blood sugar

- *Estrogen and progesterone:* regulate fertility via your menstrual cycle

- *Testosterone:* regulates sex drive and motivation

- *DHEA:* contributes to vitality

Ideally, the stress response is followed by the relaxation response, in which our heart rate returns to normal, our muscles relax, and our mind becomes calm once again. Our *autonomic nervous system* (the part of the nervous system that controls actions we don't consciously decide to take, such as breathing and heartbeat) is divided into two parts to reflect these two states. The *sympathetic nervous system* governs the "fight or flight" stress response, while the *parasympathetic nervous system* governs the "rest and digest" relaxation response, which also includes reproductive and sexual activity. You might think of the sympathetic nervous system as dominant during the day, when we're out facing challenges, and the parasympathetic nervous system as dominant at night when we're home relaxing, eating, having sex, and sleeping.

That, at least, is the healthy ideal for which our bodies were designed. But in today's busy world, with its 24-hour artificial light and its round-the-clock work schedules, our sympathetic nervous systems can be too active and our parasympathetic nervous systems not active enough. This can exhaust our adrenals, causing the stress hormones they produce to go out of balance: too high, too low, or some combination of both. As a result, we may feel "wired" (jumpy, anxious, tense, and easily upset), "tired" (fatigued, sluggish, unmotivated, unfocused), or a combination of these.

This is unfortunate because imbalanced levels of cortisol and adrenaline have powerful effects on virtually all of our other hormones. They disrupt insulin, which regulates blood sugar, along with leptin and ghrelin, which govern fullness and hunger, respectively; this has significant consequences for our appetite and our weight. Imbalanced stress hormones also disrupt our thyroid hormone, which regulates metabolism; this affects our weight, our energy, and our mood, as well as overall health.

Finally, as Lara discovered, imbalanced stress hormones disrupt our sex hormones: estrogen, progesterone, testosterone, and DHEA. This can lead to the difficulties many of us encounter with PMS, menstrual periods, and perimenopause.

Unfortunately, it doesn't take much time for your adrenals to be affected by stress but it can often take a long time for them to be restored to healthy function. In part, this is because stress and the adrenals can create a vicious cycle, as you see in the figure below.

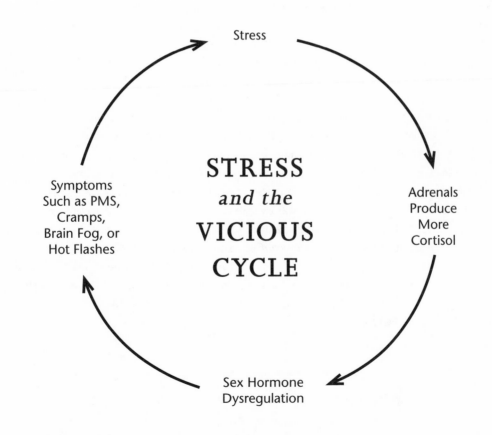

Fortunately, the reverse is also true. When you modify or remove excess stress from the system—either by changing your life circumstances, adding de-stressors to your schedule, or learning to cope with stress differently—your adrenals function better, as do all the rest of your hormones. This is what Lara found. When she reduced the amount of stress in her life, she was able to rebalance her stress hormones, which meant that her sex hormones, in turn, were also able to rebalance.

The amount of stress in our lives is often less important than how we respond to it. Changing our attitude—even slightly—can often make a huge difference in how much stress we can cope with. Our psychological response affects the way our adrenal glands release stress hormones, which has a powerful ripple effect on the rest of our hormones and therefore on the body. So figuring out how to cope with stress is one of the best things we can do for our hormones and our overall health.

Some sources of stress can also be exhilarating and pleasurable. Falling in love can be stressful, as can a romantic first date. Challenging physical activities such as hiking, rock climbing, skydiving, and the like can be thrilling *because* they are stressful; that is, they make significant demands on our minds and bodies, forcing us to rise to the occasion. Starting an exciting new job, bringing a new baby home from the hospital, embarking on a demanding creative or business project, or performing before an audience can all be stressful experiences that we choose precisely because they demand our biggest, best, and greatest efforts—the upside of stress. The high-level CEO, the Grammy-winning rock star, the world-class surgeon all embrace the stressful challenges of their chosen professions just as any of us might seek the challenges of deepening a relationship, raising a child, committing to the work we love, or contributing to our community.

However, even in these best-case scenarios, if stress is not balanced by relaxation—if both the sympathetic and the parasympathetic nervous systems do not have their say—we risk burnout in the form of adrenal dysfunction and imbalanced stress hormones. Too many stressful thrills that aren't balanced with relaxation and restful sleep might throw our entire hormonal symphony out of tune. So when women come to me with mild, moderate, or severe PMS, painful periods, or challenging perimenopause, I always make sure to look at the possibilities for modifying their stress and rebalancing their stress hormones. These are also factors I look at when women come to me with endometriosis, fibroids, or PCOS.

Some Common Sources of Stress

- Insufficient or poor-quality sleep

- Missed meals: drops in blood sugar

- Sweet or starchy meals: spikes in blood sugar

- Environmental toxins

- Unwanted, prolonged exposure to noise

- Prolonged exposure to extreme temperatures

- Illness, pain, or infection, especially long lasting or chronic

- Deadlines

- Arguments

- Emotional loss: breakup or divorce, loss of a friend

- Financial loss: loss of a job, decline of a business

- Moving

- Changing jobs or careers

- Responsibility without control

- Feeling out of control/loss of personal power

- Not enough downtime, "me time," "bliss time"

- Feelings of anxiety, depression, or despair

- Feelings of guilt, shame, unworthiness, or self-hatred

- Childhood abuse: physical, emotional, sexual

- Historical stress from families and childhood experiences

INSULIN: THE BLOOD-SUGAR HORMONE

The other major player in your hormonal symphony is insulin, a key hormone that is thrown out of balance by the typical American diet of too many sweet, starchy foods and too little protein and healthy fat. When insulin goes out of balance, you are likely to gain weight that clings stubbornly to your midsection. Excess insulin also contributes to low estrogen, PCOS, and infertility, as well as to many symptoms of PMS and challenging perimenopause, including mood swings, depression, insomnia, fatigue, acne, and migraine.

Insulin imbalance is such a common problem and so disruptive to other hormones that it's worth taking a closer look at how it develops. Here's a step-by-step description.

- **Step One:** You eat some type of carbohydrate, which is broken down into glucose, a form of sugar. The sugar travels from your digestive system into your bloodstream.

- **Step Two:** To keep your brain from getting too much sugar, which might damage your brain cells, insulin starts storing blood sugar in your body's other cells. (Insulin also alerts your liver to keep blood sugar out of the brain.)

- **Step Three:** Each of your cells has several *insulin receptors,* which function as little locks. Insulin is like the key that opens those locks, allowing it to move sugar from your bloodstream into your cells, where it is stored.

- **Step Four:** When you eat too many carbs and especially too much sweet, starchy food, eventually your cells fill up to capacity. At that point, they shut down some insulin receptors in a process known as *insulin resistance.* Meanwhile, the insulin imbalance sets off alarm signals in the form of *inflammation,* which causes a cascade of other health issues.

- **Step Five:** When cells shut down their insulin receptors, your pancreas produces more insulin, trying to overcome the resistance. Now we've set in motion another vicious cycle: more insulin leads to fewer receptors, which leads to more insulin, which leads to still fewer receptors, and so on.

- **Step Six:** When insulin can't get into your cells, it remains in your blood, a condition known as *hyperinsulinemia.* Now your blood sugar moves into your fat cells, which expand—and you start developing fat deposits around your midsection. That weight will be very difficult to lose unless you reverse your insulin resistance.

- **Step Seven:** At some point, even your fat cells won't accept any more sugar, so the blood sugar remains in your bloodstream, at which point you have developed Type 2 diabetes. You can potentially reverse or at least minimize this disorder, however, by reversing insulin resistance.

What Is a Carbohydrate?

- Grains: whole grains, processed grains, flour, corn and corn products

- Processed sugar

- Starchy vegetables

- High-glycemic fruits

- Dairy products contain both protein and carbohydrates (milk sugars)

As you can see, you want to reverse insulin resistance and restore *insulin sensitivity:* your insulin's ability to move blood sugar into your cells and use it there. At that point, your fat cells will stop expanding, and, eventually, they will even start shrinking as your body starts using insulin more efficiently. You'll lose weight, regain your body's true shape, and feel more energized, sexy, and alive. Balancing your insulin helps your body to balance other hormones as well—including testosterone, which also helps you feel sexy, sensual, and womanly.

So how do you balance your insulin and restore insulin sensitivity?

Basically, you want to build muscle instead of fat, because muscle cells have many more insulin receptors. And how do you build muscle? Through exercise plus a diet with the right amounts of protein and healthy fats, as you'll see in the 28-day plan.

To balance your insulin, you also want to reduce your carb intake and focus on *low-glycemic carbs* that are less likely to produce high blood sugar. As you eat fewer sweets and high-glycemic carbs, your body will use up some of that stored sugar in your fat cells, shrinking them. Eventually, you will have more muscle, less fat, and balanced insulin levels.

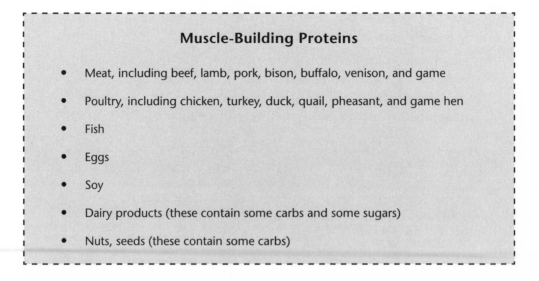

Muscle-Building Proteins

- Meat, including beef, lamb, pork, bison, buffalo, venison, and game

- Poultry, including chicken, turkey, duck, quail, pheasant, and game hen

- Fish

- Eggs

- Soy

- Dairy products (these contain some carbs and some sugars)

- Nuts, seeds (these contain some carbs)

I know this is difficult to take in because we tend to be so frightened of fat, but the true secret to weight loss for many of us is not reducing fat. It's reducing carbs while making sure to consume enough protein and healthy fats to balance our hormones, build muscle, support brain function, and maintain our energy. It's also making sure that at least half of our plate is filled with brightly colored vegetables.

Of course, you have to eat both fat and protein in moderation. If you overconsume either one, you'll gain weight. But a healthy balance of carbs, fats, and protein is ultimately your best recipe for health. This way, your body uses up its stored sugar, your cells reactivate their insulin receptors, and you finally have nice, balanced insulin levels. As a result, you will restore harmony to your hormonal symphony.

OVERCOMING PCOS AND INSULIN RESISTANCE: SHANTI'S STORY

Shanti was a web designer in her late 20s who came to see me with irregular periods, debilitating PMS symptoms, and weight gain that was frustrating her to no end. "I don't eat that much, and I exercise every day," she told me. "Yet I keep gaining weight! It's making me crazy!" Shanti was also frustrated by a persistent case of acne and by hair that had started to grow on her face and breasts. "It's so embarrassing!" she told me. "I hope you can make it stop!"

High-Glycemic Carbs That Throw Your Insulin out of Balance

- Processed sugar

- Baked goods

- White flour, pasta, bread

- White potatoes

- White rice

- Corn

- Sweet fruits, including mango, papaya, watermelon, banana

Low- and Medium-Glycemic Carbs
That Help Balance Your Insulin

- Brown rice

- Sweet potatoes

- Green leafy vegetables: spinach, kale, chard, collards, escarole, mesclun, arugula, watercress, lettuce

- Cruciferous vegetables: broccoli, cauliflower, cabbage, Brussels sprouts

- Onions

- Low-glycemic fruits: berries

- Medium-glycemic fruits: apples, pears, citrus fruits

I noticed that the weight Shanti was complaining about seemed to have concentrated around her waist, so that it was almost as wide as her hips. Together with the other symptoms she described, this was the classic profile of polycystic ovarian syndrome, a condition usually set off by insulin resistance and marked by high levels of testosterone.

Of course, I had to test Shanti's hormone levels to be sure, and the results confirmed my suspicions. Shanti's readings showed insulin resistance, while her sex hormone levels indicated high levels of testosterone and an imbalanced ratio of luteinizing hormone to follicle-stimulating hormone, two hormones crucial to regulating the menstrual cycle.

I'm always excited when people come to me with this particular problem because I know I can help them quickly. I suggested to Shanti that she take a medical food like Ultrameal 360, or chromium, while following my 28-day plan; this would balance her blood sugar and help restore healthy insulin sensitivity. Once her insulin levels were balanced, her other hormone levels would fall into place and her symptoms would clear right up.

Shanti didn't like the idea of giving up desserts, white rice, and her morning oatmeal with brown sugar, but she loved the idea of losing weight, having easy periods, clearing her skin, and losing the unwanted hair growth. So she threw herself into the 28-day plan with enthusiasm—and was rewarded with quick results. After a month, her symptoms had eased considerably and within three months, they were all gone.

"You'll probably need to follow this plan for life," I told her on her last visit. "Otherwise, the insulin resistance will return, triggering your symptoms all over again. But as long as you eat the right balance of proteins, carbs, and healthy fats, you can look forward to regular periods and a smooth transition into menopause."

Shanti's experience is a typical example of how many seemingly unrelated symptoms—acne, weight gain, hair growth, irregular periods, and PMS symptoms—can all stem from the same hormonal imbalance. It's also a beautiful illustration of the power of diet, supplements, and lifestyle to balance hormones and restore health.

THYROID: THE METABOLISM HORMONE

Thyroid regulates your metabolism, which has a huge impact on your weight, your energy levels, and your moods. When stress hormones go out of balance, your thyroid is often affected, too, which in turn triggers PMS, menstrual and perimenopausal symptoms, and other health issues.

Thyroid-induced symptoms include weight gain, constipation, hair loss, sluggishness, fatigue, depression, and mood swings. One of the first things to try is balancing your stress hormones and your insulin levels. If that doesn't work, your health-care practitioner may also recommend thyroid-supportive supplements, herbal and nutritional remedies, or medication. All of this will have a beneficial effect on your sex hormones.

FAT BEHAVES LIKE A HORMONE-PRODUCING ORGAN

Another factor that could be throwing your hormones out of whack is excess body fat. That's because body fat actually produces hormones; key among these are *cytokines,* which contribute to inflammation. Inflammation is a risk factor for cardiovascular disease, diabetes, and cancer. It also contributes to obesity. So here we have another vicious cycle: obesity produces inflammation, which in turn creates more obesity.

Another way excess body fat can disrupt your hormonal balance is by storing estrogen.

Fortunately, you can reduce excess body fat with a healthy eating plan, as well as exercise, sleep, and stress relief—all key components of weight loss. The 28-day plan in the second part of this book can help.

KEEPING YOUR HORMONAL SYMPHONY IN TUNE

Now that you've seen how stress and diet affect your hormonal balance, we can move on to the next chapter to consider specifically how to balance your all-important sex hormones.

CHAPTER 3

BALANCING YOUR
SEX HORMONES

My patient Mandy was suffering from perimenopausal symptoms: menstrual cramps, hot flashes, weight gain, and nonstop irritability. I worked with her to change her diet—removing sugar, dairy, and gluten (you'll find out why in Chapters 4 and 5) and making sure she ate more protein—and bumped up her exercise a bit more. I also suggested she use over-the-counter progesterone cream to improve her hormonal balance.

The results were immediate—and amazing. Mandy's cramps disappeared, she no longer had any hot flashes, she lost weight, her sex life improved, and she generally felt calmer. She also began thinking seriously about a career change she had long considered but had never found the courage to make.

"I think I'm finally ready," she told me on our last visit. "It's time." I loved seeing how resolving the hormonal imbalance had freed Mandy to become braver and clearer about the path that was right for her. Aging can bring wisdom, especially when we can clear away the distracting symptoms of perimenopause and menopause!

In the previous chapter we saw how balancing stress hormones, thyroid hormone, and insulin are crucial to creating overall hormonal balance. Now let's zero in on sex hormones and learn how to balance them.

ESTROGEN, PROGESTERONE, TESTOSTERONE, AND DHEA: THE SEX HORMONES

Two of the major hormones that shape your sexual feelings and your sexual identity are estrogen and progesterone. Two others, believe it or not, are testosterone—usually thought of as a male hormone—and DHEA, which is responsible for vitality, energy, and a sense of well-being. When these four hormones are in balance, everything works well: your menstrual cycle, your transition into perimenopause, your sex life, and your feelings of sensuality and pleasure. When these four hormones are out of balance, you're far more likely to struggle in all those areas.

It's nearly impossible to make progress with these four hormones if your stress hormones and insulin levels are not in balance, so if you're facing challenges with PMS, painful periods, perimenopause, sexuality, or sensuality, you'll want to address them, too.

ESTROGEN AND PROGESTERONE: THE FEMALE HORMONES

It's not quite accurate to call these "female" hormones because men have them, too, while women have their share of testosterone, the so-called male hormone. We women need testosterone for our sex drive and motivation as well as for energy and to build muscle mass. It's therefore a central part of our female identity, and we'll be looking at it more closely below. However, the menstrual cycle, pregnancy, and the transition into perimenopause and beyond are governed largely by estrogen and progesterone, the section leaders of this part of the hormonal symphony. The interaction between these two hormones, along with luteinizing hormone and follicle-stimulating hormone, directs all the different changes that take place throughout the month:

- The creation of a new layer of *endometrium,* the tissue that lines the uterus

- Maturation of the follicle that holds the egg

- *Ovulation,* by which the egg leaves the ovary and becomes available for fertilization

- Fertilization: when this happens, the egg is implanted in the endometrium; when it doesn't, the endometrial layer sloughs off, resulting in your period.

A healthy menstrual cycle lasts approximately 28 days but it can vary quite a bit. This cycle is timed to the changing moon, an ancient connection we still don't fully understand but that can be a source of power, creativity, and balance (for more on this relationship, see www.womentowomen.com/menstruation/menstrualcycle.aspx). On the first of the 28 days, estrogen levels begin to increase and rise gradually for two weeks, peaking midcycle. Then they taper off, just as progesterone starts to rise to its own peak on days 21 to 23. So for you to be hormonally healthy—to remain fertile and to avoid PMS, cramping, and perimenopausal symptoms—estrogen and progesterone need to be in balance with one another.

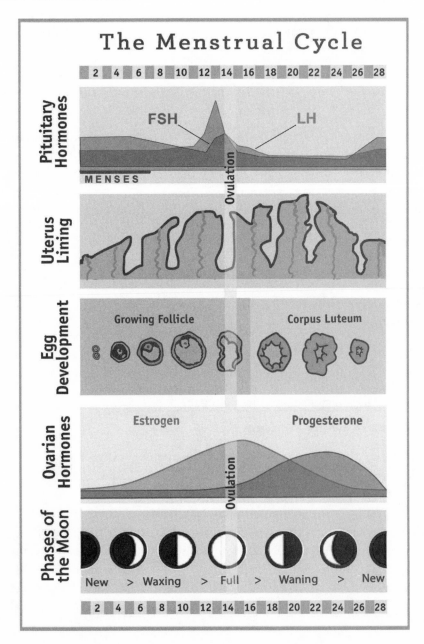

The most common way for estrogen and progesterone to fall out of balance is a condition known as estrogen dominance, in which there is simply too much estrogen *relative* to the amount of progesterone. Sometimes, we can restore balance by lowering estrogen levels; at other times, we boost progesterone levels; we can also alter levels of both. Keeping these two hormones properly balanced is nearly impossible, however, if stress hormones and insulin are not properly balanced as well.

EXCELLENT ESTROGEN

Estrogen keeps your skin soft and supple. In the right amounts, it supports mood, sexual health, and energy. Estrogen keeps you moist, not just in your vagina and genital area but all over. Dry skin might be a sign of too little estrogen, as might dry eyes.

Estrogen protects against cardiovascular disease and in the right amounts it also fights inflammation, a problematic immune-system response associated with numerous disorders including heart disease and cancer. Estrogen's anti-inflammatory properties are welcome any time but especially as we age.

In addition, estrogen is involved with body weight. This is why it's easier to gain weight and harder to lose it after hysterectomies, and during perimenopause and menopause.

The relationship between estrogen, weight, and inflammation is complicated and somewhat contradictory:

- Fat cells produce estrogen

- Fat cells create inflammation

- Inflammation contributes to weight gain

- Estrogen is anti-inflammatory

Your best ways to resolve this issue are to maintain a healthy weight and to create healthy levels of estrogen—not too high, not too low, and in the right balance with progesterone. And once again, balancing stress hormones and insulin is the best way both to maintain healthy estrogen levels *and* a healthy weight.

Although estrogen plays a big role in sexual desire and fertility, we have estrogen receptors everywhere in the body. Estrogen is also involved in memory, healthy sleep, and maintaining pain-free joints. Estrogen also affects neurotransmitters, the biochemical messengers in the brain that influence energy, mood, and focus. When their estrogen levels are too low, women come into my office feeling "frazzled," "unbelievably irritated," and "anxious" during the week or so before their periods. And when women in perimenopause tell me, "I can't think clearly" or "my attention is just *off,*" these symptoms also reveal that their estrogen levels are in decline.

On the other hand, too much estrogen in combination with low progesterone is associated with depression. This is why many girls start struggling with depression prior to menses and why women with PMS often struggle with depression as well.

I'm sharing this information with you because I want you to understand the power of your hormones and to learn to listen to what your body is telling you. But I also want you to hear the good news: many of these problems can be resolved through diet, herbs and supplements, exercise, sleep, and psychological support, occasionally complemented with bioidentical hormones. Your hormonal symphony may be playing out of tune, but balancing your hormones is well within your reach—and you can make a terrific start in just 28 days.

THE THREE FACES OF ESTROGEN

Estrogen is actually a generic name for a type of hormone. Your body has not one type of estrogen but three: *estrone, estradiol,* and *estriol.* Each behaves differently.

- **Estradiol:** This is the form of estrogen that we have in the greatest quantity. It's also the most powerful. Estradiol levels begin to decline during perimenopause, however, and decline further after menopause. That is why, in some cases, bioidentical hormone replacements can be beneficial—to continue the protective effects of estradiol. (For more on bioidentical hormones, see Chapter 5.)

- **Estrone:** Our bodies naturally produce estrone in an amount that is approximately 10 percent of our total estrogen. However, estrogen replacement preparations such as Prempro and Premarin, which are made from urine taken from pregnant horses, contain higher amounts. This is why some people are concerned about the effects of these estrogens as opposed to bioidentical estradiol preparations, which tend to have a less potent effect.

- **Estriol:** This form of estrogen also usually constitutes about 10 percent of our total, although it predominates during pregnancy. Estriol is also far less potent than both estradiol and estrone. As a result, we often use it as a vaginal cream for estrogen support, as has been done in Europe for years.

ESTROGEN METABOLISM: THE GOOD, THE BAD, AND THE UGLY

You might have heard that higher levels of estrogen in your system can potentially contribute to hormonal cancers, including breast and uterine cancer. But I have some exciting news to share with you. Cutting-edge research reveals that it isn't the estrogen levels themselves that are of concern: it's the particular pathways through which your estrogen metabolizes.

This is some of the most thrilling medical news to appear in a long time: now that we understand more about how estrogen is metabolized, we can actually influence which pathway it goes down—which means we can play an enormous role in protecting ourselves from female cancers.

I am convinced that the information I am about to give you and the suggestions I'll offer about how to decrease your risk of female cancers will become standard among health-care providers within the next 10 to 15 years. Meanwhile, almost no one is talking about this except for integratively trained medical practitioners—but the science is all there. For example, the cutting-edge research of Dr. Eleanor G. Rogan offers groundbreaking possibilities for preventing cancers. So let me share with you this game-changing breakthrough in women's health.

It all starts with the liver, which helps filter out or metabolize anything in the blood that the body can't absorb. One of these elements is estrogen. As a result of that process, we are left with *estrogen metabolites,* which are waste products left over after estrogen has been metabolized.

These metabolites differ depending on which of three possible metabolic pathways the estrogen goes down. I think of these pathways as "the good, the bad, and the ugly" because one of them results in metabolites that protect against breast cancer while the other two result in metabolites that increase your risk of breast cancer. The three possible pathways are *2-hydroxyestrone* (the good); *16-alpha hydroxyestrone* (the bad), and *4-hydroxyestrone* (the ugly). Ideally, all of our estrogen would metabolize along "2" rather than "16" or "4."

Unfortunately, some of us have a genetic predisposition to metabolize along a pathway that's less than ideal. My own body, for example, tends to choose "4"—not great news for my health. But the good news—and it's very good news indeed—is that all of us, even those of us with a problematic genetic code, can affect the pathway that our liver chooses by taking supplements, changing our diet, and making some lifestyle changes.

Your Recipe for Healthier Estrogen Metabolism

Diet

- Increase your intake of cruciferous vegetables: broccoli, cauliflower, and Brussels sprouts

Herbs and supplements

Take all of the following supplements to promote healthy estrogen metabolism

- A probiotic, one capsule taken before each meal: 10 to 25 billion mixed bacteria per capsule

- Indol-3-carbonyl: one tablet per day

- Calcium d-glucarate: one tablet per day

- Flaxseed or chia seed: two tablespoons per day

- Soy: 40 to 60 mg per day

- Turmeric: 600 mg two times per day

- N-acetylcysteine: 600 mg one or two times per day

- Resveratrol: 250 mg per day

- EPA/DHA fish oil: 2000 mg per day

- Vitamin D: 1000 to 2000 IU per day*

* Have your vitamin D tested and if it's low, work with a practitioner to find out how much to take.

Detox

- Decrease toxins in your environment (for more on this, see Chapter 6)

- If necessary, work with a practitioner to detoxify your body

Especially helpful in supporting healthy estrogen metabolism is reducing stress in all its forms: psychological, physical, and environmental. High levels of adrenaline and cortisol can increase the amount of estrogen that travels down the two less healthy pathways, as can high concentrations of pesticides and toxins.

Another obstacle to healthy estrogen metabolism is digestive difficulty. If you are suffering from constipation, diarrhea, bloating, or gas, this might be a sign of a digestive problem such as yeast overgrowth, parasites, food sensitivity, insufficient healthy bacteria in your gastrointestinal tract, or small intestine bacterial overgrowth. Any of these conditions can make it very difficult to metabolize estrogen correctly. You also need to have one or two bowel movements every day to move excess estrogen out of your system. (For more on how to improve digestive health, see Chapter 5.)

So your best defenses against "the bad and the ugly" are diet and exercise, herbal supplements (see the box on page 45), resolving any digestive issues, and reducing both environmental and psychological stress (which we'll learn more about in Chapter 6).

Now that you have this most recent information, you can make a huge difference in your own hormonal health. And if you have digestive issues that don't easily clear up with diet modification and the addition of a probiotic, please see a practitioner who specializes in this area.

POWERFUL PROGESTERONE

Progesterone is a very calming hormone. Many women who don't realize they are progesterone deficient struggle with such symptoms as anxiety, irritability, and moodiness, which can become so intense that it can feel like your body has become host to an alien invader. Progesterone deficiency can also lead to PMS, abdominal weight gain, extremely heavy periods, and spotting between periods. In fact, progesterone is crucial in the timing of your cycle, so if you don't have enough, you may have difficulty with your menstrual rhythm. In the worst-case scenario, insufficient progesterone leads to buildup of the menstrual lining, which poses the risk of uterine cancer.

The good news is that when I help my patients balance their progesterone levels, they feel a renewed sense of health and vitality. If they have previously suffered from progesterone deficiency, they also feel at peace in a way they've never experienced before.

Don't Forget the Progesterone!

If you are taking estrogen and you have a uterus, please be aware that you should also be taking progesterone to counterbalance the estrogen's effects. Estrogen causes the uterine lining to thicken, while progesterone helps it to slough off. Taking estrogen without progesterone means that your uterine lining becomes thicker and thicker. If you are not sloughing off the tissue, you put yourself at risk for developing hyperplasia, which can become uterine cancer.

Luckily, progesterone can protect you. Just be mindful that you never take estrogen without its protective partner. Progesterone by itself is okay; estrogen by itself is not.

TESTOSTERONE: THE SEX DRIVE AND MOTIVATION HORMONE

Although we think of this as a male hormone, testosterone is actually crucial to our female identity. The challenge is to keep it in the proper balance with estrogen and progesterone. Too little and we feel unsexy, unmotivated, and possibly depressed. Too much and we might end up with hair in the wrong places *(hirsutism),* excessive anger and irritability, and other hormonal problems.

Women who are insulin resistant tend to have more testosterone, so overcoming insulin resistance can be helpful in bringing their testosterone down into balance. On the other hand, insufficient testosterone can make it difficult to build the muscle mass that helps decrease insulin resistance. So once again, it's a symphony, with every player affecting every other.

Recently, a trend has emerged of prescribing testosterone to women in their 40s, 50s, and beyond to increase their vitality and sex drive. I would rather see you increase your testosterone naturally, which gives you the greatest chance of keeping your hormones in balance. Too many practitioners simply prescribe testosterone without taking the entire hormonal symphony into account. However, testosterone *can* be remarkably helpful, so if you can't increase your supply naturally, taking additional testosterone in consultation with your practitioner may be the right choice.

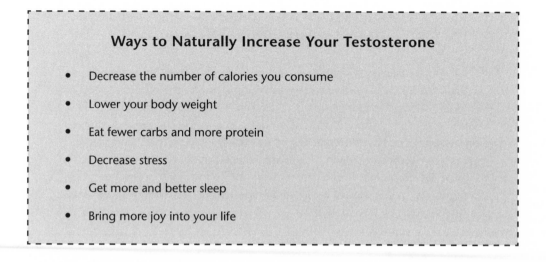

Ways to Naturally Increase Your Testosterone

- Decrease the number of calories you consume

- Lower your body weight

- Eat fewer carbs and more protein

- Decrease stress

- Get more and better sleep

- Bring more joy into your life

DHEA: THE "FEEL-GOOD" HORMONE

This hormone has a remarkable effect on people's ability to deal with stress, repair their bodies, increase lean body mass, and help with weight loss. It also works to decrease insulin resistance, supports immune and brain function, and generally improves well-being and vitality.

When you are DHEA deficient, you tend to have low energy and feel irritable. You may also suffer from stiffness in the joints. Once again, healthy adrenals and balanced stress hormones help support your DHEA production. I sometimes prescribe DHEA, especially when I am helping patients overcome adrenal dysfunction or insulin resistance. DHEA can also be useful during perimenopause, as it increases supplies of testosterone, estrogen, and progesterone; restores libido; and helps with such symptoms as brain fog, memory issues, and anxiety.

Pregnenolone: Mother of the Sex Hormones

The hormone precursor to many sex hormones is *pregnenolone*. Many practitioners seek to restore hormonal balance by prescribing pregnenolone, which certainly has a lot of potential benefits. I personally prefer supplementing with DHEA because I've had such fantastic results with it, but pregnenolone is another viable choice.

PERIMENOPAUSE: YOUR TRANSITION INTO MENOPAUSE

When we first start menstruating, our estrogen-progesterone balance is geared toward the biological goal of reproduction; it continues to be throughout our 20s and 30s. As we move into our 40s, our bodies begin to prepare for the stage when childbirth and child rearing will not be our biological focus. This stage, known as perimenopause, ends with menopause, when our periods stop and our ability to get pregnant ends.

Once again, it's not just our sex hormones that make this transition. Our cortisol levels go up, creating additional problems with stress and hormonal disruption. So finding ways to modify stress becomes increasingly important as we get older. We also become more prone to insulin resistance during perimenopause, which means that maintaining a healthy diet and appropriate exercise becomes increasingly important as well.

Before menopause, most of our estrogen is made in our ovaries. As our ovaries become less active, the balance shifts, until finally, during menopause, about 50 percent of our body's estrogen and progesterone is being made in our adrenals. If our stress levels are high, however, our adrenals won't "waste" any resources on making estrogen or progesterone: they'll focus on making the stress hormones that we need for the fight-or-flight response. Modifying stress will help ensure us an adequate supply of estrogen in our 40s and beyond.

As your ovaries start making less estrogen, your body looks elsewhere for this crucial hormone. Since one key source is fat cells that store estrogen, your body might start creating more fat cells. This can give you access to more estrogen, but it also means you'll gain weight. If you're already obese when you begin perimenopause, those extra fat cells might create too much estrogen relative to your progesterone, which would require you to increase your progesterone levels.

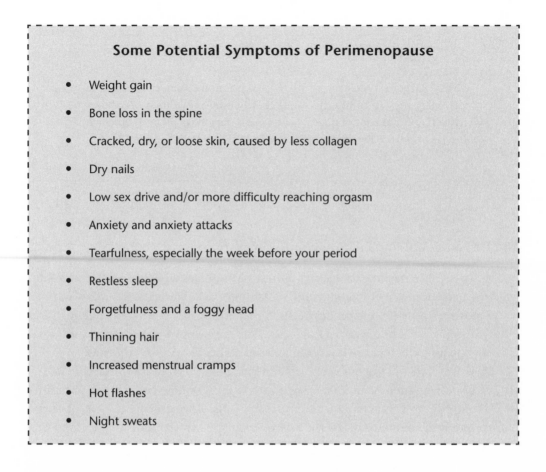

Some Potential Symptoms of Perimenopause

- Weight gain

- Bone loss in the spine

- Cracked, dry, or loose skin, caused by less collagen

- Dry nails

- Low sex drive and/or more difficulty reaching orgasm

- Anxiety and anxiety attacks

- Tearfulness, especially the week before your period

- Restless sleep

- Forgetfulness and a foggy head

- Thinning hair

- Increased menstrual cramps

- Hot flashes

- Night sweats

ENJOYING YOUR HORMONAL SYMPHONY

As you've seen, your hormonal symphony includes many different instruments, each of which affects the other. Keeping the whole symphony working in harmony may seem like a daunting task, but I promise you, it's not! As you move into Chapter 4, you'll find out how to let go of what doesn't work so you can focus on what does.

CHAPTER 4

LET GO OF WHAT
DOESN'T WORK . . .

Michelle was a homemaker in her 20s with a toddler and an infant. "I love my kids," she said to me on her first visit. "But right before my period, I feel like I'm the worst mom in the world. I scream at the kids like a crazy person and then I feel bad afterward. I don't want to be like this! I try not to be so short-tempered, but no matter how hard I try I can't seem to get things under control. I thought it must be my hormones but I had them tested and the doctor said they were normal. He offered to put me on the birth-control pill, but I was on it during college and I used to get these awful headaches. I didn't want to mess with it again. There *must* be something wrong with me—but what?"

Michelle went on to describe the rest of her symptoms. "Some months, I get so much bloating that I have to wear different-size pants," she told me. "I'm just ravenous around that time of the month, too—I can't stop eating junk food even though I know I shouldn't. I feel worn out during the day, but at night I'm wide awake and I can't get to sleep no matter what."

For much of the month—not just before or during her period—Michelle felt groggy during the day, so she relied on coffee and diet soda to keep herself going. "I start mainlining caffeine first thing in the morning and keep going right through dinner time," she told me. "At least the coffee helps keep my appetite down. Otherwise, I'd be hungry all the time!"

It certainly sounded as though Michelle might be suffering from hormonal imbalance. I knew I'd have to test her to be sure, but meanwhile I wanted to rule out other potential conditions she might have, including anemia, thyroid issues, depression, or a viral or bacterial infection. I also wanted to hear more about her diet and lifestyle.

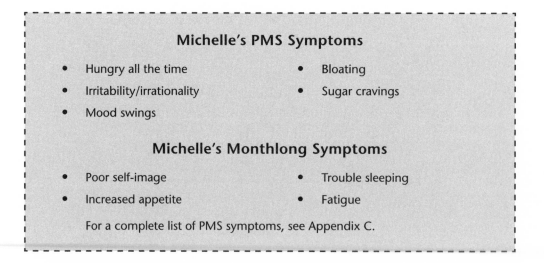

Michelle's PMS Symptoms

- Hungry all the time
- Irritability/irrationality
- Mood swings

- Bloating
- Sugar cravings

Michelle's Monthlong Symptoms

- Poor self-image
- Increased appetite

- Trouble sleeping
- Fatigue

For a complete list of PMS symptoms, see Appendix C.

Like many mothers of small children, Michelle was constantly on the go, with very little time for herself. She told me she averaged about five hours of sleep each night, and when I asked her about exercise, she just laughed. "The only exercise I get is running after my kids," she told me. "When do I have time to do anything else?"

Michelle told me that she had gained 40 pounds since she started having children. Feeling horrible about the way she looked, she skipped meals whenever she could. She almost never had breakfast, shared a peanut-butter-and-jelly sandwich on white bread with her toddler for lunch, and usually made a big, starchy family dinner. She wanted to provide good food for her family, but she also needed to stretch the budget as far as possible. After a stressful day, Michelle usually found it impossible to resist joining her husband in eating cake, cookies, and ice cream after dinner.

Like most young mothers, Michelle was leading a fairly high-stress life. She worked a few afternoons a week at her local post office, leaving her children with her sister. She was also active in her church. Her husband worked two jobs so she saw very little of him—usually just a rushed dinner and maybe a hectic weekend morning. Michelle felt that she had very little time for anything fun, including sex with her husband—"which I *used* to enjoy!" she said with a sigh.

I had a working hypothesis about what might be going on with Michelle's hormones, but of course I couldn't be sure without more information. So I gave her a saliva test that measured the stress hormones produced by her adrenals—a take-home test requiring her to take samples at four points during the day: morning, midday, evening, and bedtime.*

---

* In some cases, adrenal hormone readings are so extreme or adrenal symptoms are so severe that Addison's disease or Cushing's syndrome might be involved. These two forms of adrenal

I also gave Michelle a blood test to evaluate her insulin levels after she had fasted for 12 hours. Then I had her eat a very sweet, starchy meal (I usually suggest pancakes with syrup) and took a second blood test two hours later. Looking at the two levels would give me more information about whether Michelle was insulin resistant.

In addition, I checked Michelle's levels of thyroid hormone, which regulates metabolism. I sometimes run a blood test to evaluate sex hormone levels as well, looking at estrogen levels on day 3 of a woman's cycle and at progesterone levels on day 25. Alternatively, I might do a saliva test for sex hormones on day 25. Either way, I also make sure to test for DHEA and testosterone, as well as the levels of *sex hormone binding globulin* (SHBG), a carrier protein in the blood that binds to testosterone and estrogen. If your SHBG is high, you don't have access to your testosterone or estrogen even if absolute levels of those hormones are high, so I want to check that out as well.

Finally, I gave Michelle a urine test to measure her neurotransmitters, which help determine mood, mental focus, and energy. Together these tests gave me a snapshot of what was going on with Michelle's stress hormones, thyroid hormone, sex hormones, and neurotransmitters.

As I had suspected, they were all significantly out of balance.

Tests for Hormonal Imbalance

- Adrenal stress index/saliva test, taken four times in a day, to measure cortisol, adrenaline, and other stress hormones

- Fasting insulin and two-hour postprandial (after a meal) insulin test, the first test taken after fasting and the second taken two hours after a high-sugar, starchy meal, to measure insulin sensitivity

- Thyroid tests: TSH, free T3, free T4, thyroid antibodies, reverse T3, and total T3

- Blood or saliva test to measure the three estrogens, progesterone, testosterone, DHEA, and SHBG

- Urine test to measure neurotransmitters (epinephrine, norepinephrine, gamma-aminobutyric acid [GABA], serotonin, glutamate, histamine, and dopamine), the hormones that control mood, focus, and energy

---

dysfunction go beyond the conditions described in this book, and require a very different form of treatment.

THE STRESS MESS

Imbalanced stress hormones are at the root of just about every type of problem with PMS, periods, and perimenopause, as well as having a significant effect on the hormonal issues of endometriosis, fibroids, PCOS, and premature ovarian failure. As I had suspected, Michelle's stress hormones were significantly out of balance.

Stress hormones are supposed to be at their highest levels when you wake up in the morning—in fact, they actually *wake* you up—and then gradually taper off during the day. But Michelle's hormones were low in the morning and high in the evening. Furthermore, these out-of-balance stress hormones were playing havoc with the rest of her hormones. For example, Michelle's thyroid tested on the low end of normal (remember, thyroid function can be disrupted by imbalanced levels of cortisol and adrenaline). Most conventional practitioners might not have considered that score a problem, but I thought that low thyroid might be slowing Michelle's metabolism, contributing to her weight gain and occasional low mood.

As happens with so many young mothers, Michelle's life was one long round of obligations, demands, tasks, and deadlines. Here were some of the key stressors in her life:

- Taking care of two young children

- Maintaining the household

- Money worries

- Guilt about not doing more for her sister, who did so much for her

- Frustration with her husband, who never seemed to be home

- Not enough time for relaxation, fun, or sex

- No time with girlfriends

In addition to the emotional stressors in Michelle's life, there were physical ones:

- Not getting sufficient sleep

- Missing meals

- Blood sugar spikes and crashes caused by a sweet, starchy diet

These physical and emotional challenges were kicking Michelle's stress hormones into overdrive, pushing her sex hormones out of balance as well. Her PMS, ongoing exhaustion, sleep problems, and raging appetite were the predictable results.

IMBALANCED DIET, IMBALANCED HORMONES

Another key piece of the puzzle was insulin. Michelle's blood tests suggested that she was suffering from insulin resistance, a condition that can result from excess consumption of carbohydrates: grains and flour, sugar and sweetened foods, starchy vegetables, and fruits. When insulin can no longer move sugar into the cells, the insulin level in the blood rises. This creates a host of health problems, disrupting both the stress hormones and the estrogen-progesterone balance.

Michelle's diet contributed to insulin resistance in two ways. First, she skipped breakfast and ate only a couple of times during the day. As a result, her blood sugar levels dropped when she missed meals and then spiked suddenly when she ate a big, starchy meal or had a sweet snack. This threw her insulin out of balance. Second, Michelle ate a lot of foods that contained processed sugar and white flour—foods that break down quickly into blood sugar. Her insulin had trouble moving all of this sugar into Michelle's cells. When insulin levels remain high—as Michelle's did—the cells become resistant and unresponsive, refusing to allow insulin to move sugar into the cells. If you remain insulin resistant for too long, you run the risk of blood sugar levels rising in response. Since the next potential step, if the problem continued, was diabetes, I wanted to help Michelle reverse this pattern as soon as possible.

Causes of Insulin Resistance

- A diet high in sweet, starchy foods

- Not enough proteins or healthy fats

- Missing meals, especially breakfast

- Stress

- Toxicity

- Heavy metals

- Inflammation

- Persistent organic pollutants (POPs), such as pesticides and other industrial chemicals in the environment

Meanwhile, Michelle's insulin resistance was putting a strain on her system, which further imbalanced her sex hormones—and her stress hormones. At the same time, her imbalanced stress hormones were affecting her insulin levels and intensifying her insulin resistance. This was a classic vicious cycle that I wanted to interrupt.

NEUROTRANSMITTERS AND SEX HORMONES

As we've seen, neurotransmitters are the hormones and other biochemicals that govern mood, energy, and focus. When your stress hormones go out of balance, your neurotransmitters are disrupted as well. Likewise, when your blood sugar and insulin aren't properly balanced, your neurotransmitters are affected. Just think of how irritable you feel when you've missed a meal, or how calm and happy you feel when you eat something filling and nutritious. Both stress and diet play enormous roles in how well balanced our neurotransmitters are.

One key neurotransmitter is serotonin, the hormone that protects against depression, poor sleep, lack of self-confidence, and low self-esteem. Michelle's serotonin levels were unusually low. Sugar gave her temporary bursts of productive energy—but only until she crashed and the cravings intensified.

Another key neurotransmitter is dopamine, the hormone that floods our body when we undergo a thrilling experience such as a roller-coaster ride, an exhilarating mountain hike, or a romantic first date. Michelle's dopamine levels tended to fluctuate wildly, so that sometimes she felt irritable and tense while at other times she felt unmotivated and spacey.

All of this hormonal disruption was in turn disrupting Michelle's sex hormones. Her estrogen registered as high-normal, while her progesterone was low-normal. Although both hormones were in the normal range, the proportions were off, creating estrogen dominance. As a result, Michelle was prone to weight gain (because of the excess estrogen), often felt jittery (without the calming effects of progesterone), and was subject to mood swings (because of the estrogen-progesterone imbalance).

As if this weren't enough, Michelle's testosterone and DHEA were both at the low end of normal. This made her feel less sexy and sensual than she once had and less motivated and energetic, as well.

FIGURING OUT WHAT DOESN'T WORK

When I went over Michelle's test results with her, she was astonished to learn that so many aspects of her life were contributing to her hormonal imbalance—and vice versa. I reminded her of the good news: it's easy to rebalance your hormones once you know what kind of diet, lifestyle, and psychological support you need. But in order to figure out what does work, it's helpful to know what doesn't. So let's look at the key elements that were disrupting Michelle's hormones:

- Sweet, starchy diet with insufficient protein and healthy fats

- Missed meals

- Too much caffeine

- Not enough sleep

- Not enough exercise

- Too much stress with not enough support

These are all common problems for the women I treat. Now let's dig a little deeper into how each of these elements contributes to hormonal imbalance.

WHAT DOESN'T WORK: A SWEET, STARCHY DIET WITH INSUFFICIENT AMOUNTS OF PROTEIN AND HEALTHY FATS

In Chapter 2 we saw how eating sweet, starchy foods overloads your blood sugar and contributes to insulin resistance. We've talked through the basic biology: by overloading your body with too many carbs, you produce massive spikes in your blood sugar levels, creating insulin surges. Although this cycle is generally unhealthy, each of us responds to it in our own way. Exercise can affect our ability to metabolize sugar and produce insulin. So can our proportion of muscle to body fat.

Genetics also plays an important role. You may remember the 2004 documentary film *Super Size Me*, in which filmmaker Morgan Spurlock spent 30 days on a fast food–only diet. In five days he gained nearly ten pounds. Soon he began to experience depression, lethargy, and headaches that could be relieved only by eating more fast food. By the end of the month, he had gained a total of more than 24 pounds and had developed heart palpitations. His girlfriend claimed that he had lost most of his energy and his sex drive.

It took Spurlock months to lose the weight he had gained and restore his health. Meanwhile, other people replicated his experiment with quite different results. Another filmmaker tried a similar fast-food diet, but she added exercise to the mix and didn't eat nearly as much as Spurlock did. As a result, she actually *lost* weight. A group of Swedish students also replicated the study in an experiment supervised by their professor. Some of these students gained weight, some actually lost weight, and some stayed the same. However, none of them suffered from the same weight gain or symptoms as were chronicled in the film.

So what do we conclude from these various responses? They underscore something I've seen countless times in my practice: we each have different responses to what we eat and how we live. For example, some of us have a dramatic response to sweet or starchy foods while others are more resilient: in other words, food speaks to our genes—and to our jeans! In addition, some of us may be more resilient when we are younger, when we exercise more, when we are getting more sleep, or when we are experiencing less stress in our lives.

However, if you are struggling with PMS, difficult periods, perimenopause, endometriosis, fibroids, PCOS, or premature ovarian failure (POF)/infertility; if you are gaining weight or are unable to lose weight; or if you are eating a high-sugar and/or high-carbohydrate diet, you can be virtually certain that your diet may be contributing to your trouble. Your food intake is speaking to your genes in ways that they just don't want.

One of my favorite sayings is "Food is information—and your best medicine." Eating a sweet and starchy diet gives your body all the wrong messages. Instead of telling your cells to remain insulin sensitive so they can continue to store sugar from the carbs you eat, you are telling your cells to become insulin resistant. Instead of telling your blood sugar to remain at nice, even levels, you are inviting it to spike and crash. Instead of instructing your insulin to remain at healthy levels, you are asking it to go out of balance. The message to your body with a sweet and starchy diet is "Gain weight, add stress to the system, and start a hormonal cascade that will create unwanted symptoms."

So if you are experiencing weight gain or struggling with hormonal symptoms, your body is sending *you* a message. It is trying to tell you that you are feeding it the wrong information—that it needs different foods to keep your hormones healthy.

WHAT DOESN'T WORK: MISSED MEALS

One of the greatest stressors on your system is going too long without eating. When you miss a meal, your insulin levels remain high as your blood sugar crashes. If this continues for a few hours, you will develop symptoms of low blood sugar: irritability, mental confusion, shakiness, anxiety, or depression. These symptoms continue until you eat, at which point your blood sugar soars.

This jagged pattern of blood sugar spikes and crashes is bad for you in several ways:

- You're likely to eat more and crave more starches and sweets as a way of quickly bringing your fallen blood sugar back up to a normal level. (Low serotonin levels also produce sugar cravings.)

- You are more likely to develop insulin resistance.

- Your blood sugar crashes stress your body, pushing your cortisol levels further out of balance.

- In a vicious cycle, the excess cortisol further imbalances your blood sugar and hormones.

- For many reasons, you're likely to gain weight: because of eating more, because of the resulting insulin resistance, and because of the excess cortisol that cues your body to hold on to weight.

- Your imbalanced stress hormones and your imbalanced insulin will likely contribute to imbalanced sex hormones, which in turn will potentially lead to PMS, painful periods, perimenopausal symptoms, endometriosis, fibroids, or PCOS.

The Yeast Factor

If you have sugar cravings, another cause might be systemic yeast, which is an overgrowth in your intestinal tract. Conventional medicine has been slow to accept the existence of systemic yeast but integrative medicine has accepted it for a long time, and there is growing support for it in the scientific literature. For more information on how to identify and clear up this problem, see my previous book *The Core Balance Diet*.

If you're not digesting your food properly, you're likely to have trouble detoxifying your estrogen, so if the 28-day plan isn't enough to resolve digestive issues, please work with a health-care practitioner who can help you.

As we'll see in Chapter 5, the answer is regular, moderate-sized meals, evenly spaced throughout the day, with your first meal taken within 30 to 60 minutes of waking. That is the most hormone-friendly choice you can make, and one guaranteed to help restore hormonal balance.

WHAT DOESN'T WORK: TOO MUCH CAFFEINE

There is so much conflicting information out there about caffeine. Is it good for you, bad for you, or both? A little bit of caffeine is probably helpful for some people. However, if you don't metabolize caffeine very well, it may be causing you problems. For most women, one or two daily 8- to 10-ounce cups of coffee or a similarly caffeinated drink is fine, preferably one. But I've seen the caffeine habit sneak up on women, particularly at midlife. As with most habits, moderation is the key, and there is no one right answer for every woman.

Caffeine really does help you feel more awake—at least at first. Brain studies show that it reduces sleepiness and improves alertness, effectively jump-starts a sleep-deprived mind, and increases the ability to pay attention. Feelings of fatigue can be offset by caffeine consumption, and when tiredness does set in and you feel less focused, it can help increase your energy levels. There is also good evidence behind the claim that caffeine improves productivity and task performance. An even more intriguing benefit may be its capacity to stimulate positive feelings and perk up your mood. And although the results of studies are mixed, moderate caffeine consumption may genuinely improve both long-term and short-term memory.

On the other hand, excessive use of caffeine might lead to problems, especially if you are caffeine sensitive or your adrenals are compromised. If you're suffering from adrenal dysfunction, caffeine is simply terrible for you because it pushes your adrenals even harder. The caffeine buzz prompts your adrenal glands to pump out more of the stress hormones cortisol and adrenaline. If you are already struggling with hormonal imbalance, caffeine might be setting off an additional cascade of hormonal problems, including menstrual and perimenopausal symptoms.

This is what Michelle found. She had become dependent on caffeine to function, which led me to believe that it was probably causing her problems. Her difficulties sleeping, her experience of fatigue, and her premenstrual symptoms all suggested that caffeine was contributing to her hormonal imbalance.

So what should *you* do about caffeine? My advice is simple:

- Limit or avoid your intake of caffeine if you are at risk for cardiovascular problems or if you have sleep problems.

- Limit or avoid caffeine if you get headaches or have other withdrawal symptoms when you miss your "daily dose"; the withdrawal symptoms are telling you that your body can't handle so much caffeine. (For help withdrawing from caffeine, see my website, www.womentowomen.com.)

- If you do indulge in caffeine, savor it! Sip your coffee, tea, or cocoa slowly, as a special treat, rather than mainlining it to keep yourself awake.

- Choose the healthiest possible form of caffeine. Tea is probably best, but high-quality coffee or chocolate can also be a healthy choice if you don't load up your caffeinated drinks with sugar or cream. Sodas—whether diet or regular—are often loaded with additives and other problematic ingredients that can make menstrual symptoms worse (see Chapter 5).

WHAT DOESN'T WORK: NOT ENOUGH SLEEP

These days, everyone is working harder. Workweeks are getting longer, people are putting in more overtime, and more and more people are working two or more jobs. A recent article by Rachel Emma Silverman in *The Wall Street Journal* blog reported that in many parts of the corporate world, the new full-time workweek is considered 90 hours, while a 40-hour week is considered part time. This means people are sleeping less—with disastrous results for their health. One of the best things you can do for any health condition is to get seven to nine daily hours of deep, refreshing sleep; one of the worst things you can do is skimp on sleep.

So when Michelle told me that she routinely got fewer than six hours of sleep each night, I worried that her hormonal imbalance and her premenstrual symptoms were at least partly the result. Inadequate sleep revs up your stress hormones, setting off the hormonal cascade that, as we have already seen, can be so harmful. As we saw in Chapter 2, our sympathetic nervous system rules during the day, gearing us up for challenging and perhaps stressful activities. We need the evening and nighttime to relax and sleep so that our parasympathetic nervous system has the chance to restore balance.

Exactly how much sleep do you need each night? Here again, each of us is different. Some of us are happy with seven hours, some of us need eight, and some of us don't feel right unless we get a full nine hours. Our sleep needs may vary depending on diet, exercise, and stress levels, so once again, listening to your body is key.

Creating good conditions for restful sleep is an important part of restoring your hormonal balance. Here are my favorite sleep tips:

- Avoid sugar, caffeine, or alcohol if you think they are interfering with your sleep.

- Eat lightly for your last meal of the day, avoiding high-fat foods that may be more difficult to digest.

- Unplug an hour before bedtime and keep electronics out of the bedroom. The bedroom is for sleep and sex! The flickering electronic light on your computer or television can cue your brain toward wakefulness, and having your computer in the bedroom can remind you of work and other stresses.

- Exercise earlier in the day, since vigorous movement within a few hours of bedtime can wake you up and keep you up.

- Be sure your room is dark and quiet and has comfortable bedding. Don't allow electronics or digital clocks to "zap" you in the night.

- Consider the herbal and nutritional supplements in the 28-day plan to ease your adrenal stress, which might also contribute to wakefulness.

WHAT DOESN'T WORK: NOT ENOUGH EXERCISE

I know it can be hard to find the time and motivation to exercise. But exercise is a crucial piece of the puzzle when you are trying to balance your hormones and improve your health.

First of all, exercise helps you make the transition between the sympathetic and the parasympathetic nervous systems. After spending a day in "stress overdrive"—meeting deadlines, caring for the kids, responding to the demands of loved ones—exercise really gives you the chance to release some anger, anxiety, and frustration and helps with the transition from "fight or flight" to "rest and digest." By lowering your stress threshold, exercise helps your adrenals produce lower amounts of cortisol and other stress hormones, which in turn helps prevent the hormonal cascades that cortisol can set off. (Be careful about exercising if you're too stressed or fatigued, as extra exertion can add to your stress and further tax your adrenals, making your situation worse. If you're exhausted after you exercise, you probably want to get your adrenals tested, as people suffering from adrenal dysfunction should not push their heart rates above 90 beats per minute.)

Exercise can also help stimulate your production of dopamine, an energizing hormone, and DHEA, one of the sex hormones that increases energy and libido. Exercise builds muscle, which is associated with increased testosterone, a sex hormone that will also help stimulate your sex drive.

When I told Michelle that failing to exercise was throwing her hormones further out of balance, she looked at me in dismay. "How in the world will I ever find time to exercise?" she asked me. "I barely have time to take a shower!"

Believe me, I get it. I'm a mother, too, so I understand how challenging it can be to find time to exercise, especially when your children are young. This, though, is one of those times when you need to put yourself first. Exercise is so important that I suggest you try to get creative. Here are some suggestions for making time to exercise:

- If you have little children at home, get one of those jogging strollers and make your cardio workout a game. Your best exercise is "bursting" for a total of about 20 minutes, four days a week. Put your kids in the jogger, say, "Okay, kids, Mommy is going to go very, very fast now!" and run as hard as you can for 30 seconds while pushing your children. Then slow down for 90 seconds, and repeat. Your children will think this is a delightful game—and you'll be getting your workout.

- With slightly older children, you can make a game of chasing and being chased. Or use an egg timer for "now we're running super-fast," and "now we're walking regular." Working out *with* your children can be a way of killing two birds with one stone.

- If you're working full time and don't have time to exercise in the evening, buy an X-iser (see Resources), a step machine that gives you strength training benefits in just a couple of minutes. Even two minutes on this wonderful device is a fantastic workout. Divide up your 20-minute workout into ten 2-minute segments, taken at odd moments throughout the day. In two minutes you won't work up a sweat, so you don't have to worry about your clothes.

I'd like to add one more personal message to you if you're struggling with too many obligations and not enough time for yourself. Believe me: I know what that's like. But think of a cup that's empty—completely drained. That's like a woman who has done so much for others that she simply has nothing left to give. Now imagine the same cup brimming with nourishment. This woman has so much more to give to herself and the people she loves—her family, friends, children, and partner.

WHAT DOESN'T WORK: TOO MUCH STRESS WITH NOT ENOUGH SUPPORT

Of all the factors that affect my patients' hormonal issues, perhaps the most misunderstood is stress. As we've seen in previous chapters, stress is not just "in your head." It's a physiological reaction that involves a massive hormonal cascade that in turn disrupts the rest of your hormones.

The fascinating thing about this response is that it doesn't distinguish between actual danger, memories of danger, and potential danger. Running away from an actual tiger, remembering a tiger attack, and imagining a tiger attack all trigger the same set of physiological responses. Whether the danger is real, remembered, or imagined, our heart races, our blood pressure rises, and our breathing speeds up, while our appetite vanishes, our stomach acids drop, and our sexual response seems to disappear.

What is really important to remember is that our bodies handle modern sources of stress—deadlines at work, worries about money, relationship problems—in very much the same way as actual physical danger. So when we're stressed by any actual, imagined, or remembered challenge—from a near miss in traffic to an angry boss—we trigger that response, which always begins with our adrenals releasing a cascade of stress hormones.

When we need to rise to the occasion—whether to flee from a mugger or meet a deadline—we're very grateful for this hormonal cascade. But when our stress response goes off too often, when we can't turn it off, or when we feel as though most of our days are lived in unremitting stress, we have a problem. At this point we are facing genuine health risks to our heart, our cardiovascular system, and our immune system (stress suppresses our immune reaction). And of course, all those stress hormones flooding our system play havoc with the rest of our hormones—including our sex hormones.

Our bodies are built to handle one-time emergencies, whether it's a late night, a major deadline, or a week spent taking care of a sick child. We have more difficulty with prolonged stress unrelieved by relaxation or restoration. That's the situation so many of my patients are in: the hormonal cascade set off by their prolonged stress disrupts their hormones and well-being on multiple levels, contributing significantly to their health problems.

This was certainly Michelle's situation. From the moment her baby woke her up in the morning until the moment she lay down to sleep at night, she felt as though she was always on the go, always on call, always faced with demands that were just a little too much for her to meet. Because the demands were unrelenting, she never really knew how to turn off that "stress alert" response. As a result, her system was almost continually flooded with stress hormones.

Coping with continual stress in the present was challenging enough. But there was another dimension of Michelle's stress that further complicated the picture. Michelle was also dealing with stress from the past.

Historical Stress

Sometimes the sources of our stress have more to do with echoes from the past than with situations in the present. By the time Michelle was four, she had three younger siblings. Michelle's mother was overwhelmed by her situation, and Michelle vividly remembered the constant crying of babies whose diapers had not yet been changed.

Michelle also remembered her mother's periodic explosions of rage. "You're no help at all!" Michelle's mother would yell at her four-year-old daughter. "Don't you see what a hard time I'm having? Why don't you do something to help me instead of making more trouble?!"

Afterward, Michelle's mother was apologetic and tried to comfort Michelle. But to Michelle, these outbursts were terrifying and she tried to be "the best little girl in the world" in hopes of avoiding them. She learned to take care of herself, and she tried to suppress all the anxiety she felt about making a mistake, creating more problems, or making life harder for her mother.

This anxiety came with a price, of course, because from a very young age, Michelle was carrying an enormous amount of stress. First, she continued to put a lot of effort into being "good," not bothering others, and fending for herself: efforts that were frequently stressful. Then, whenever she saw anyone in a rage—a customer yelling at a waitress or a mother at the park scolding her children—Michelle felt some of the same terror she had felt as a child.

To make matters even more challenging, Michelle found herself repeating her mother's pattern with her own children. The guilt and shame she felt after "losing it" with them only added to her stress.

Outwardly, then, Michelle behaved like a calm, competent mother. Inside, though, she often felt like a terrified little girl. These anxieties added another layer of stress to Michelle's situation, helping to keep her "stress alert" permanently on. If Michelle was going to rebalance her sex hormones, she would need to calm her stress hormones first.

I've written more fully about this concept in *Is It Me or My Adrenals?* There I describe three ways to modify stress:

1. Daily "stress busters": a bath, a quiet cup of tea, a quick walk in the woods, or any other activity that gives you pleasure and relief from stress for even as little as five minutes at a time. (See the 28-day plan for a list of five-minute stress busters you can try.)

2. "Stress-release" practices, such as yoga, tai chi, or meditation. Numerous studies have shown that these can be remarkably effective in dissolving stress and developing resources to meet life's challenges. (You can find more information on these approaches in Appendix D.)

3. Mind/body approaches to address historical stress, including art and dance therapy; Emotional Freedom Technique; Byron Katie's "The Work," and the Hoffman Institute's Quadrinity Process. (You can learn more about these in Appendix D.)

MAKING TIME FOR STRESS RELEASE

When I talked with Michelle about the possibility of coping with her current and historical stress, she looked at me as though I were crazy. "I barely have time to be here now, talking to you!"

"I really understand," I told her. "But let's see if we can find some things that you do have time for—just a few minutes can make a big difference. Let's try to come up with a plan that will work for you."

One tool I've found very helpful is the emWave, a little device that gives you immediate feedback on your heart rate. Placing your thumb onto the emWave machine can be your reminder to breathe, slow down, and relax—even for just one or two minutes. (For more information, see Resources.)

Another possibility is to meditate for just two minutes at a time, twice a day, and work up to five to ten minutes. Close your eyes, breathe deeply, and try to empty your mind—for just 120 seconds. Taking that tiny bit of time to release tension before, say, moving clothes from the washing machine to the dryer, can make a surprisingly big difference in your overall stress levels. Going outside for a walk with the kids has a calming effect, too, and it teaches them the value of spending time outdoors. We must always remember that the lasting impressions we make on our kids come from what we do, not from what we say they should do.

Another creative solution that I used to rely on was arranging a playgroup with other young mothers I knew. Sometimes just being with other grown-ups helps reduce stress for moms, especially while the children are young. Sometimes you can trade off so that each woman gets a couple of hours to do something for herself. Perhaps you can pool resources to find a low-cost sitter through your local college or university.

Here is my best suggestion for busy women, with or without children: take a few moments right now to shut your eyes and ask yourself, *If I had a free two hours, what would I like most?* If two hours seems like too much to imagine, ask yourself what you would like for an hour, or half an hour. Then see what comes to mind. Is it time by yourself, with a friend, or with your romantic partner? Do you want to read, take a bath, go for a walk, see a movie, or have a fabulous cup of coffee in a local café? Imagine what weekly treat would make you feel happy and relaxed—and then see what you can do to work toward it.

INSUFFICIENT TREATMENTS

Throughout this chapter I've suggested ways to let go of what doesn't work: a sweet, starchy diet, missed meals, lack of exercise, insufficient sleep, and excessive stress, including historical stress. I also want to suggest letting go of the insufficient treatments that most conventional practitioners commonly prescribe: antidepressants and birth control pills.

Antidepressants

I'm all for antidepressants if a woman is moderately or severely depressed and needs biochemical support to balance her neurotransmitters. Even in that case, though, it's remarkable how much progress many women can make with diet, exercise, herbs, nutritional supplements, and the psychological support they need.

Antidepressants can be less effective for mild depression, let alone for hormonally induced mood swings. A recent study claimed that for treating mild depression (as opposed to moderate or severe depression), antidepressants were no more effective than placebos! Yet far too many practitioners are influenced by the pharmaceutical industry, which sends armies of sales representatives to "educate" practitioners about the virtues of a particular medicine.

I can see why in some cases antidepressants might be effective. Most antidepressants that are prescribed for hormonal issues are SSRIs, selective serotonin reuptake inhibitors. This type of antidepressant basically keeps more serotonin in your system, enabling you to benefit from this key hormone. Serotonin combats depression, builds self-esteem and a positive outlook, and creates feelings of calm. It also supports healthy sleep. Clearly, having access to increased supplies of serotonin can be terrific when you are struggling with PMS, painful periods, or perimenopause.

However, SSRIs don't help rebalance your stress hormones and they don't address the diet, lifestyle, or psychological issues that contributed to your stress in the first place. Furthermore, hormonal imbalance isn't just a mood issue. If you suffer from estrogen

Natural Remedies for Depression

If you have been diagnosed with bipolar disorder or if you are currently taking an antidepressant of any kind, check with your health-care practitioner before taking any of these supplements.

- Fish oil EPA/DHA: 1000 to 2000 mg per day

- Vitamin D: 1000 to 2000 mg per day

- Folic acid: 400 mcg per day

- 5-HTP, a precursor to serotonin: 50 to 150 mg at night *or* L-tryptophan, a precursor to serotonin: 250 to 1000 mg per day

- Theanine: 200 to 250 mg per day

- Tyrosine: 500 to 1000 mg per day

dominance, as Michelle did, you are at risk for numerous health problems. I want you to be in glowing health throughout your life—through perimenopause, menopause, and beyond. If antidepressants make you feel well enough to cope with your life stresses and make some key changes, I'm all for them. But if your practitioner uses them to mask the hormonal issues, I'm concerned because I want to be sure that the underlying problems are solved and that your potential hormonal dangers are overcome.

After all, no one ever got depressed because they were suffering from a "Prozac deficiency." Depression is a complicated condition that is at least partly set off by hormonal imbalance. Rebalancing your hormones and restoring hormonal health is the most important thing you can do to combat your depression. So before you start the antidepressants, try the 28-day plan in the second part of this book, which will help combat mild depression as well as hormonal imbalance.

Birth-Control Pills

If a woman chooses birth-control pills to enable her to have an active sex life while avoiding the risks of pregnancy, that might be a wise choice. But we still don't fully understand how "the pill" affects a woman's body. We only know that it takes over a woman's ovarian function, so that her body does not produce its own hormones and instead depends on the pill to supply them. We don't really know anything about the long-term effects of suppressing ovulation, which is worrisome to many of us in health care.

For this reason, I prefer other ways of treating hormonal issues that I consider safer, healthier, and more effective. As with antidepressants, the pill only masks the underlying imbalance problem rather than addressing it.

If You Are Taking the Pill . . .

Be sure to supplement with vitamin B and a good multivitamin. The pill contributes to lower levels of vitamin B and other nutrients, so make sure to keep restoring your body's nutritional reserves to a healthy level.

MICHELLE'S SOLUTION: A WORK IN PROGRESS

Like many of my patients, Michelle was initially overwhelmed by the thought of all the changes I was asking her to make. I reassured her that she could make these changes at her own pace—or not at all. The important thing was that she understood how her body worked and what her options were.

The first suggestion I made was that she start eating more frequently: three meals and two snacks evenly spaced throughout the day, with her first meal taken within an hour of waking up. That would help balance out Michelle's blood-sugar levels, combating insulin resistance. Eating more protein and healthy fats while cutting back on the sweets and starches would also go a long way toward achieving those goals.

Exercise would help both with insulin resistance and stress relief. So would getting sufficient restful sleep.

Finally, looking at the sources of stress in her life would make a huge difference for her. Like most of us, Michelle faced a triple task:

- Modify the stresses she faced

- Build some more pleasure and "me time" into her day, her week, and her month

- Uncover the historical sources of her stress—and then, if necessary, take further action

While this was all a lot to take in and to think about changing, Michelle was relieved to know that there were solutions. And she found it empowering to know that she *could* make these changes, which *would* improve her health, her mood, and her life. "I like knowing that I don't have to depend on anyone else to fix this," she told me on her second visit. "There is a lot that *I* can do!"

Michelle started slowly, just cutting back on sweets and making an effort to start the day with a high-protein breakfast. When she saw what a difference this made to her mood, energy, and PMS symptoms, she decided to give my full 28-day plan a try. She found a 20-minute workout routine she could do four times a week while her children napped (see Resources for some suggestions) and discovered that exercising made her feel both more calm and more energized. She and her husband also found a sitter to take the children one morning each weekend, giving the couple a few hours together.

The changes Michelle made paid off quickly. Within 28 days of going on my plan, she experienced significant relief. By the third month she told me, "I feel like my old self again!"

Michelle is still figuring out how to modify the stress in her present life while continuing to explore ways of releasing historical stress. But knowing there is a solution, as she puts it, "makes all the difference in the world." We'll look further at that solution in the next chapter.

CHAPTER 5

... And Start Doing What Works

Chantelle was a 47-year-old marketing executive who, until recently, had felt a real sense of satisfaction in her life. The mother of two college-age children, she had been enjoying the newfound freedom of not having her kids at home. She and her second husband enjoyed a solid second marriage that had just passed the five-year mark. Chantelle had also started work at a new firm. She told me, "After a lifetime of paying my dues, I feel like I am finally getting the respect and appreciation that I've always wanted. And frankly, I think I deserve it!"

Chantelle also had a warm circle of friends and a close relationship with her younger sister, and, after years of fighting, she felt that she and her mother were finally getting along. "I've come so far in my life," Chantelle told me on her first visit. "But *what* is going on with my body?"

Despite all the good things in her life, Chantelle was having a very rocky perimenopause. With no changes in her diet or exercise regimen, she had gained 20 pounds in the past year and was frustrated by symptoms that she didn't understand: memory problems, mental fog, fatigue, and a complete loss of interest in sex.

"Sex? What's that?" she said when I asked her about her sex life. "That's not even on my radar these days! Joe and I had been looking forward to having the house to ourselves with the kids gone . . . but now I can't even get interested!"

Chantelle was also having some hot flashes and occasional night sweats, sometimes during her period but sometimes in the middle of the month. Even when she didn't have night sweats, she was having difficulty sleeping. If she did fall asleep, she often woke up in the middle of the night, her mind racing, her heart pounding.

"I'm tired all the time," she told me. "And I never used to have trouble sleeping, no matter how worried I was about money, or work, or the kids, or whatever. Now I'm really not worried about anything—and yet I can't sleep! It doesn't seem fair."

Chantelle was a classic example of how hormonal imbalance can create a difficult perimenopause, even when life circumstances are very good and life stress is relatively under control. "I spent years working too hard," Chantelle admitted to me, "but I've finally figured out how to take time for myself and enjoy life. But with this weight, and the not sleeping, and the no sex, and the hot flashes, I *can't* enjoy my life and everything I was looking forward to."

When I asked about her diet, Chantelle shook her head.

"I don't understand why I can't lose weight," she told me. "I eat so healthy! For breakfast I have a granola bar. For lunch I just have a plain salad—not even any dressing! For dinner, maybe some whole-wheat pasta or some brown rice and veggies. But I can't lose any weight at all!"

I asked Chantelle what she did for exercise, and again she shook her head. "I go to the gym for a spin class," she told me, "and I'm taking yoga, and I recently added some weight training. Wouldn't you think with all of that I'd be losing weight? But instead, I'm gaining. And not muscle, either, but fat—right around my belly. How can this be?"

I told Chantelle that she seemed to be coping with several different types of hormonal imbalance but that I needed to test her before I could be sure. Indeed, Chantelle's tests revealed hormonal imbalance in a number of areas: her stress hormones, insulin levels, and sex hormones. Until she rebalanced her hormones, she would find it nearly impossible to lose weight, no matter how little she ate or how much she exercised. Fortunately, now that we understood the problem, I could help Chantelle achieve hormonal balance. She actually needed to eat both differently and more.

HORMONES OUT OF BALANCE

Unlike Lara, whom we met in Chapter 2, Chantelle's hormonal imbalance seemed to have less to do with life stress and more to do with hormonal shifts that often accompany the transition from fertility to menopause. In a way, this was good news because it meant that when I offered Chantelle the herbal remedies I usually prescribe for perimenopause—a combination of black cohosh, red clover, wild yam, and chasteberry—she would likely find that many of her symptoms cleared up right away. (For more on specific suggestions for perimenopause, see page 236.)

Sources of Hormonal Imbalance

- Ongoing life stress

- Ongoing "attitude stress," such as feelings of guilt, shame, anxiety, confusion

- Ongoing historical stress, in which feelings in the present are intensified because of experiences from the past

- A high-carb diet without sufficient protein or healthy fats

- Excess body fat

- Missing meals, or too much time between meals

- Chronic exposure to toxins in air, food, water, and household products

- Insufficient sleep

- Perimenopause

If you're eating a hormone-friendly diet, getting good sleep and exercise, and getting the psychological support you need to cope with stress, you may be able to sail through perimenopause. Even then, however, you may need herbal, nutritional, or hormonal support. And if your hormones are already imbalanced, perimenopause can be the extra challenge that produces a host of new problems, including Chantelle's symptoms of exhaustion, mental fog, memory problems, loss of sex drive, and weight gain.

However, age wasn't the only issue. Chantelle's diet was also stressing her system with too many carbs and not enough protein or healthy fats. A granola bar might sound healthy but it's really little more than a candy bar—a very sweet, starchy snack that metabolizes into sugar very quickly. By starting her day with something sweet, Chantelle was cuing her metabolism to begin a pattern of blood sugar spikes and crashes that imbalanced both her insulin levels and her stress hormones.

Chantelle's lunchtime salad might have been a healthy choice if she had added some lean, high-quality protein (chicken, beef, fish, nuts, seeds, or goat cheese) and some healthy fats (olive oil, flaxseed oil, or walnut oil). But a plain salad with no dressing is actually not nourishing enough by itself. We need to include protein and fats in every meal or snack to maintain a healthy blood-sugar level.

Her evening meal posed the same problem. Moderate amounts of whole-wheat pasta or brown rice might be healthy choices but only if they're accompanied by protein and healthy fats. In addition, pasta contains gluten, to which many people are sensitive. Gluten sensitivity can create a whole new set of stresses on your system, leading to additional hormonal imbalance.

Chantelle was also waiting far too long between meals. To maintain steady levels of blood sugar and healthy insulin levels, you want to eat small meals or snacks every three to four hours, with some protein and some healthy fat in every meal or snack.

Chantelle's lack of sleep was causing still more problems. Although your body can adapt to an occasional night of short sleep, you want to be sure to get seven to nine hours at least five nights out of seven—and seven nights out of seven is even better. Her stress hormones were being thrown off by insufficient sleep, which in turn contributed to imbalance in both her insulin levels and her sex hormones. The herbal remedies I prescribed would help reestablish that balance. Meanwhile, I suggested some natural sleep aids that could help Chantelle sleep until that happened. (See the box entitled "Natural Sleep Aids" on page 90.)

I explained all of this to Chantelle. Then I suggested that she follow my 28-day plan: a healthy diet, appropriate supplements, moderate exercise, and restful sleep. If the plan didn't work, I told her, we might consider some bioidentical hormones. But Chantelle wasn't ready to make so many changes.

"Honestly, I'm just overwhelmed," she told me. "I probably *should* do all these things you're talking about. But I just don't think I can."

"I understand," I told her. "And I know I'm asking a lot. But if you can manage this approach, your health will improve, you'll feel more optimistic, and you'll have more stamina. As you begin to make these changes, they get easier and easier. And the payoff is huge!"

"I'm sure you're right," Chantelle said again. "I just don't think I can do it."

"Then let's start slowly," I suggested. "Doing the whole plan gives you the best results. But even a few small changes can make a huge difference."

"Okay," Chantelle agreed after a moment. "Let's start slowly."

Chantelle started out with "Plan A" (see box on opposite page). She cut sweet and starchy foods out of her diet, replacing her granola bar with a protein shake that included two tablespoons of ground flaxseed or chia seeds. She took the supplement N-acetylcysteine and stopped using plastics in her microwave. All of these factors helped her metabolize estrogen in a more healthy way. She added some chicken or fish to her lunch and dinner, increased her intake of vegetables, and took my recommended supplements every day. She was surprised at what a difference even those few changes made. She began to feel both more calm and more energized as well as more hopeful and confident about the future.

After a month, Chantelle decided she was ready to try my whole plan. She felt the benefits immediately. Eating a hormone-healthy diet, getting good sleep, and taking the herbal remedies I prescribed helped Chantelle tap into new reserves of energy, stamina, and hopefulness. These hormonal changes enabled her to cope with stress differently and rebuild her physical and emotional resources. To her great relief, she also began losing weight.

"I feel clearer, stronger, and happier," she told me. "It's hard sometimes to make sure I eat first thing in the morning and to stick to your three meals plus two snacks—sometimes it's just a lot of work eating that often! But it's such a relief to finally lose weight!"

Chantelle's experience is a good example of what happens with many of my patients. Although you get the best results from following my entire 28-day plan right from the start, you may not be able to make so many big changes so quickly. You may need to move into a hormone-healthy diet and lifestyle step by step.

That's fine. Do the steps that work for you, do them at your own pace, and don't give up. You may be satisfied with the results of these initial changes and choose to stop there or they may give you the strength and the motivation to go further. Either way, I'll help support you as you make the changes that are right for you.

Two Approaches to My 28-Day Plan

Plan A:

- Eliminate sugar and sweet foods from your diet

- Increase your daily intake of colorful vegetables

- Take my recommended supplements (see pages 136–138)

- Stop using plastics in your microwave

Plan B:

- Follow my 28-day plan

FIGURING OUT WHAT WORKS

What *does* work to improve hormonal health? The solution is surprisingly simple—and effective:

- **Eat a hormone-healthy diet:** quality lean proteins, organic as often as possible; plenty of fresh fruits and vegetables; and a reduced intake of carbohydrates. When you do eat carbs, make sure they're gluten free, low glycemic, and high fiber: sweet potatoes, brown rice, quinoa, or gluten-free pasta. Make sure that at every meal, half your plate is made up of colorful, nonstarchy vegetables. Avoid sugar, refined flour, junk food, artificial sweeteners, additives, preservatives, high-fructose corn syrup, and trans fats. Eat small, evenly spaced meals and snacks.

- **Identify food sensitivities:** Food allergies can be dramatic and severe, but many women struggle with hidden food sensitivities they're not even aware of. Freeing your body of this burden will help restore hormonal health. The most common food sensitivities are gluten, dairy (sometimes goat- and sheep's-milk products are okay), eggs, and peanuts. Some people have difficulties with corn and soy.

- **Move your bowels once or twice a day:** See my suggestions elsewhere in this chapter for improving digestive health. If they don't work, consult a health-care practitioner.

- **Take hormone-healthy supplements:** A good multivitamin, fish oil, the right herbs, and some other key nutrients can help balance your hormones.

- **Get sufficient sleep and exercise:** This is crucial for hormonal health and rebalancing.

- **Every day, find some quiet time to connect with nature and/or spirit:** This is especially important if your life is on overdrive.

- **If the rest of the plan doesn't give you all the results you want, consider bioidentical hormones:** Bioidentical hormones resemble those in your own body more closely than more commonly prescribed hormones do. (For example, the more commonly prescribed versions of estrogen are made from the urine of pregnant mares.) Bioidentical progesterone can be extremely helpful with severe PMS symptoms and with easing the transition into menopause.

Let's take a closer look.

WHAT WORKS: FOLLOW A HORMONE-HEALTHY DIET

Throughout this process, one of the things that surprised Chantelle most was how profoundly her diet affected how she felt. When she started the day with a granola bar and didn't eat again until that salad at lunchtime, she felt wired, spacey, and grouchy. When she started the day with a high-protein smoothie, had a snack at 10 A.M. of almond butter and an apple, and then added grilled chicken, walnuts, and a lemon–olive oil dressing to her salad at lunch, she felt calm, energized, and optimistic. To her delight, even though she was eating more food, she was finally able to lose weight.

"Supporting my blood sugar levels puts me on an even keel," Chantelle told me enthusiastically. "I feel like a different person!"

I was happy to hear this but it didn't surprise me. There are solid biochemical reasons why diet affects our stamina, mood, energy, and focus:

- **Protein** gives us the amino acids we need for brain function while helping keep our blood sugar stable.

- **Healthy fats** contain the essential fatty acids we need for both brain function and hormone building.

- **High-fiber, low-glycemic carbs** (sweet potatoes, brown rice, or gluten-free pasta) break down into sugar far more slowly than low-fiber, high-glycemic carbs (white potatoes, white rice, regular pasta). As a result, we feel full and satisfied all day long, avoiding the blood sugar spikes and crashes that stress our systems and create insulin resistance.

- **Fiber** also helps with digestion, which leaves us feeling lighter and freer as we eliminate more toxins from our body and metabolize our food more efficiently. To get enough fiber, make sure you sit down to a plate that is half full of colorful vegetables.

Eating a healthy, lean-protein diet generally leaves us with more energy and stamina, while supporting our neurotransmitters with the right vitamins, minerals, proteins, and healthy fats improves mood, energy, focus, and sleep. Balancing our hormones through diet also improves our sex drive, as well as feelings of being sexy and sensual. Generally, the right diet helps us burn calories, create lean muscle, bring down excess levels of estrogen, and increase levels of progesterone, leading to a healthy hormone profile. And remember that creating lean muscle increases overall metabolic function, which is great both for balancing our sex hormones and for losing weight.

ATTENTION: VEGETARIANS AND VEGANS

My colleagues and I agree: our vegetarian and vegan patients often find it difficult to maintain good hormonal health and healthy weights on this diet. It's difficult to stabilize your blood sugar and your insulin long term when you're eating only vegetable protein, and all too often carbs become the go-to choice.

A vegetarian or vegan diet also means you must be extremely careful when choosing your sources of protein and combining different foods to get complete proteins. My patients often start out eating a healthy vegetarian or vegan diet but then start slipping. Before they know it, they end up with debilitating fatigue and other serious symptoms—all of which clear up almost immediately once they add a little fish or chicken to their diets.

"I hate you—and I feel great!" one of my patients said to me recently. "I *loved* being a vegetarian, and I didn't want to stop. But I've felt so terrible for so long—and as soon as I started eating fish the way you told me to, I started feeling terrific. I just can't argue with that."

So, if your principles allow it, please add some fish or another type of animal protein to your diet. If you are deeply committed to remaining completely vegetarian or vegan, take extra care to do it carefully and smartly. Be sure to get vigorous, muscle-building exercise to help balance your insulin levels, and if you're not willing to take fish oil, then supplement with flaxseed oil to get the essential fatty acids you need for your neurotransmitters and hormones.

Finally, if you're on a vegetarian or vegan diet, be mindful that vitamin B12 deficiency is rampant in that population—and you need B12 for your hormonal health. So please take 1000 mcg of sublingual B12 per day.

WHAT WORKS: HAVE AT LEAST 25 TO 30 GRAMS OF FIBER EVERY DAY

Dietary fiber is the indigestible portion of plant foods, also known as "roughage." Although there are no nutrients in fiber, it helps move food through your digestive tract, improves your elimination, and pulls toxins and excess fat from your system. Fiber lowers cholesterol and makes a huge contribution to weight loss.

Most Americans don't get nearly enough fiber but it is one of the best weight-loss secrets I know, as well as one of the most important components for improving hormonal health. Remember when we learned about the importance of metabolizing estrogen down the proper detox pathway in the liver? As you'll recall, encouraging estrogen to metabolize along the correct pathway is crucial for avoiding female cancers (breast and uterine) as well as some male cancers, including prostate. Fiber is one of the key elements that direct estrogen down those healthy pathways.

In addition, hormonal balance depends upon your liver efficiently metabolizing estrogen, which is then eliminated through your bowel movements. Ideally, you would move your bowels once or twice each day, because if this detox-and-elimination process isn't working well, your estrogen levels can rise, throwing your hormones out of balance. Fiber assists with both detox and elimination, helping you metabolize estrogen in the healthiest possible way and balance your hormone levels.

If you follow my 28-day plan, you'll get all the fiber you need. For other sources of fiber, see the box below entitled "Fabulous Fiber." And please be sure to consume at least two tablespoons a day of flaxseed or chia seed—perhaps in your smoothies or on your salad. You need these ingredients to help direct your estrogen along the healthiest possible metabolic pathways.

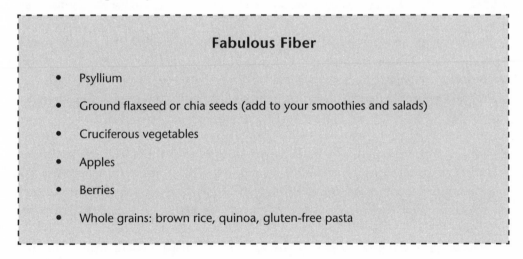

Fabulous Fiber

- Psyllium

- Ground flaxseed or chia seeds (add to your smoothies and salads)

- Cruciferous vegetables

- Apples

- Berries

- Whole grains: brown rice, quinoa, gluten-free pasta

WHAT WORKS: EAT LOTS OF CRUCIFEROUS VEGETABLES

Cruciferous vegetables or "crucifers" get their name from a form of the word "cross"; when you cut them open, you can see their cross-shaped core. Crucifers include broccoli, cauliflower, cabbage, and Brussels sprouts. This type of vegetable is high in sulfurofane, a key nutrient that encourages your estrogen to metabolize down the correct pathway in the liver.

These types of vegetables are also rich in other nutrients. If you have trouble eating several servings a week, you can throw some broccoli or cabbage into a smoothie and drink it for breakfast. Depending on what other ingredients are in there, you won't even taste it!

WHAT WORKS: EAT SEVEN TO TEN DAILY SERVINGS OF COLORFUL VEGETABLES, ORGANIC IF POSSIBLE

The more deeply colored a vegetable is, the more dense the nutrients are likely to be, so you want as much color as possible on your plate. Brilliant red peppers, deep purple eggplant, dark-green kale and collards, orange carrots, and bright-yellow summer squash are all wonderful sources of vitamins and other key ingredients. Most Americans eat two or three servings of vegetables each day, but I'd like you to get that number up to seven, or even ten.

Both organic and conventionally grown vegetables have about the same nutrients, so in that sense, both are equally good for you. However, organic vegetables have three important advantages.

First, they taste better! So do organic meat and chicken—you can tell the difference right away.

Second, they don't contain pesticides, which, as we will see in Chapter 6, can add significant stress to your system, potentially raising your cortisol levels and beginning a hormonal cascade that could ultimately worsen your symptoms. Moreover, pesticides can function as *xenoestrogens;* that is, they mimic the effects of estrogens or they can block hormonal pathways. Either way, they potentially contribute to hormonal imbalance.

Third, organic vegetables have a special strength that they will share with you, which is why I'd love you to go organic. Think about how organic plants need to fight off insects in their environment. When you consume them, you assimilate some of their ability to withstand stress. The scientific term for this quality is *hormesis,* which means "a generally favorable response to stressors." Unfortunately, foods grown with fertilizers and pesticides don't have that same quality.

So go organic—and add as many vegetables to your diet as you can. I promise you will feel the difference within a month or two, if not sooner.

WHAT WORKS: GREEN TEA, POMEGRANATES, AND ARTICHOKES

All three of these items help direct estrogen metabolism down the correct pathway in the liver, which, as we have seen, contributes greatly to hormonal health by promoting breast health, decreasing your risk of female cancers, and reducing the symptoms of fibroids and endometriosis.

WHAT WORKS: EAT SMALL, EVENLY SPACED MEALS AND SNACKS

This is one of those areas where you might hear different experts offering different kinds of advice. Some people counsel eating every three hours, while others say every four to six. You might hear the suggestion to eat three meals plus two snacks or to eat five to six small meals a day. (It's still a good idea to have a long period of fasting overnight.)

This is one of those areas that, in my opinion, is completely individual. Some people only need to eat three meals a day and don't seem to show any ill effects from eating slightly larger meals and no snacks. Listen to your body and do what works for you, which is always a good idea in any event.

That said, if you are suffering from adrenal issues, with symptoms such as fatigue, sluggishness, or an overreliance on caffeine; if you are insulin resistant; if you are diabetic or hypoglycemic; or if you are finding it difficult to lose weight, almost certainly you need to lower your intake of carbohydrates and make sure to eat five times a day: three meals plus two snacks. Your symptoms are evidence that you need a steady supply of protein throughout the day to support your energy, mood, and focus.

Whatever your ultimate decision, you will surely benefit from eating within an hour of waking up—ideally, within half an hour. If you aren't hungry first thing in the morning, consider a breakfast smoothie containing high-quality protein and some healthy fat in the form of flaxseed or chia seeds.

It's also important that each time you eat, you include some protein. Having just a piece of fruit, some carrots, or a plain salad will challenge your insulin and trigger your stress hormones. We're all under so much stress these days that I see more people than ever with blood sugar dysregulation. We all need protein! Adding protein to your snacks helps balance your blood sugar and your insulin, feed your brain, and keep you feeling calm. Including some healthy fats each time you eat will also help with insulin balance and hormone building.

Like many people, Chantelle found it challenging at first to alter her mealtime rhythm. She was used to eating only three times a day, and she considered it good for weight loss to skip a meal if she could. (In fact, skipping meals actually causes you to gain or retain weight if you do it often.) When Chantelle and I talked about this, I explained to her that waiting too long to eat breakfast and skipping meals throughout the day puts the body into "starvation mode." Our bodies evolved so they could stretch resources when food was scarce, which is why much of our physiology is designed to conserve body fat. Missing or even delaying a meal cues your body to slow down your metabolism, especially if you do so frequently. You also stress your system, which raises your levels of cortisol; and cortisol, in turn, cues your body to retain fat.

If, like Chantelle, you find it difficult to create a new eating rhythm for yourself, I urge you to follow my 28-day diet plan, even for a single week. Give yourself a few days to follow a regime of small, frequent meals and allow your body to get used to this new approach to food. You are likely to discover both that you feel more energized *and* that you're losing weight.

Food and Your Genes

You might have heard a lot about how genes determine many aspects of your health, your hormones, and even your personality. However, new research indicates that although we can't yet change our genes, we can affect how they express themselves. Diet, herbs, supplements, exercise, sleep, and even psychological support can all have an enormous influence on which of our genes step onto center stage and which remain quietly in the background.

This is amazing news! It means that even if you have a genetic predisposition to certain conditions—for example, diabetes—the right diet and lifestyle can often cue your problematic genes to remain silent so you can successfully avoid your genetic risk. Regardless of your genetic inheritance, you can have enormous power over your own health.

WHAT WORKS: AVOID SUGAR AND ARTIFICIAL SWEETENERS IN ANY FORM, INCLUDING BAKED GOODS, ICE CREAM, AND REGULAR OR DIET SODAS

Believe me, I know how good sugar can taste! But it is such a problematic and addictive food choice that I'd like to steer you away from it as much as possible. A little sugar probably won't hurt you now and then, but it's almost impossible to hold your sugar intake to "a little sugar." For most people, eating an occasional sweet snowballs into eating the whole container.

Contrary to popular belief, this is *not* a question of willpower. Your brain responds to sugar much the way as it does to cocaine and heroin, so it makes sense that your body feels like it can't get enough. And, like cocaine and heroin, sugar doesn't do your body any favors! As we've seen, sweet foods throw your blood sugar out of balance and contribute to insulin resistance, which quickly leads to weight gain. Imbalanced hormones disrupt your thyroid (which regulates metabolism) and your sex hormones (which, among other things, regulate your sex drive and your feelings of sensuality). So next time you're tempted by a sweet treat, remember how unsexy it can make you feel!

In his book, *Diet Rehab,* psychologist Mike Dow cites a March 2010 study by The Scripps Research Institute showing that rats who were fed high-fat, high-sugar diets of bacon, sausage, chocolate, and cheesecake developed neurochemical dependencies that might be described literally as "food addictions." These rats actually suffered from withdrawal-like symptoms when they were deprived of their sweet, high-fat diet—which is often the experience my patients describe.

Sugar triggers many feel-good brain chemicals, to which some people have a much stronger response than others. If you are one of these people, it may be even harder for you to resist sugar. Either way, the sugar high you feel really does serve as a kind of temporary antidepressant, as psychiatrist Henry Emmons, M.D., says in his book *The Chemistry of Joy.* Unfortunately, the effects of sugar never last long, and then you start looking for another fix. I encourage you to choose longer-lasting and healthier forms of satisfaction.

Artificial sweeteners also make it difficult to lose weight because they interfere with the body's ability to associate sweetness with a high-calorie food. This is called *calorie dysregulation*, and it explains how you can keep eating long after your body has had all the calories it requires. Restore your natural sense of hunger and fullness by avoiding both real sweeteners (including honey) and artificial ones. The three exceptions are stevia, xylitol, and erythritol, all of which are natural ingredients that don't seem to alter your blood-sugar levels nearly as much as other sugars, which makes them safe to use as you will.

Sugar Plus Caffeine: A Dangerous Combination

One of the worst things you can do for your hormone balance is to load your caffeinated drinks up with sugar. The combination of sugar and caffeine sends your adrenal glands into overdrive, flooding your body with stress hormones and contributing to weight gain, insulin resistance, and hormonal imbalance.

WHAT WORKS: IDENTIFY FOOD SENSITIVITIES

Food sensitivities are surprisingly common—and frequently misunderstood. When I first told Chantelle that I wanted to test her for food sensitivities, she was confused. "I don't think I'm allergic to anything," she told me. "I've always been able to eat whatever I wanted."

I explained to Chantelle that food *allergies* are one type of immune-system reaction, in which the body responds to otherwise harmless foods as though they were dangerous invaders. When this happens, immunoglobulin E—a type of antibody that plays a large role in allergies—mobilizes the body's resources against the foods, creating immediate symptoms such as hives, rashes, swelling, a scratchy throat, and, in extreme cases, difficulty breathing. Food *sensitivities,* by contrast, are also an immune-system reaction but they involve less aggressive antibodies. These symptoms may be delayed for hours or even days, making them much harder to detect. For a look at potential symptoms, see the box entitled "Some Symptoms of Food Sensitivity" on page 87. Both food allergies and food sensitivities differ from a third condition known as *lactose intolerance,* which is *not* an immune-system reaction but simply the result of the lack of an enzyme needed to digest lactose, a sugar found in milk and dairy products.

While a food sensitivity won't put your life at risk, it can play havoc with your hormonal health as well as your weight and overall health. Food sensitivities also create the immune-system reaction of inflammation. If you're already struggling with PMS, painful periods, or perimenopause, food sensitivities can give you a double whammy.

You have three options here. An integrative practitioner can test you for food sensitivities with a simple blood test. You can also go to the Resources section and find a practitioner who can test you. Or you can cut out some of the most common "trigger" foods for three weeks and see if you feel better. Many people have hidden sensitivities to gluten (found in grains and baked goods), dairy products (especially those made with cow's milk; products from goats and sheep may be okay), eggs, and peanuts. Soy and corn are also challenging for some people, as are citrus and berries. Try pulling some or all of these foods from your diet and see what happens. If your skin clears up, your energy increases, and your mood brightens, you may do better without those foods, at least for a while. Sometimes eliminating the food eliminates the sensitivity so every three to six months you can try reintroducing problem foods and see if any of your symptoms come back.

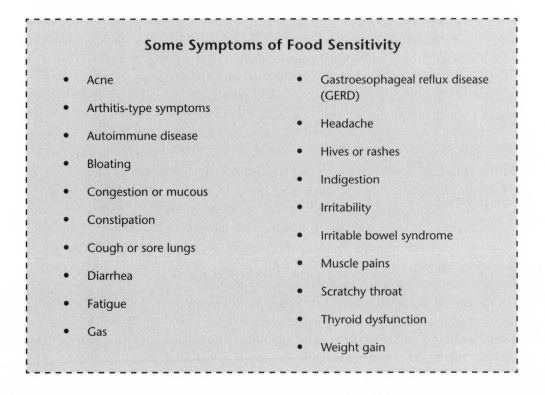

Some Symptoms of Food Sensitivity

- Acne
- Arthitis-type symptoms
- Autoimmune disease
- Bloating
- Congestion or mucous
- Constipation
- Cough or sore lungs
- Diarrhea
- Fatigue
- Gas

- Gastroesophageal reflux disease (GERD)
- Headache
- Hives or rashes
- Indigestion
- Irritability
- Irritable bowel syndrome
- Muscle pains
- Scratchy throat
- Thyroid dysfunction
- Weight gain

WHAT WORKS: TAKE HORMONE-HEALTHY SUPPLEMENTS

My 28-day plan includes suggestions for all the basic supplements you need (see pages 136–138). Even if you don't follow the entire plan, I urge you to add the supplements to your daily routine. A good multivitamin is key to your hormonal health, particularly if, like most people, you're not able to eat 100 percent organic. Conventionally grown food is not always so dense in nutrients, which means you probably need to take supplements.

If you've taken the birth-control pill at any point in your life, you are especially likely to be nutrient deficient, particularly in B vitamins. Stress also depletes vitamin B, zinc, and magnesium. If you're sensitive to dairy and pull it from your diet, you may not be getting enough calcium. Supplements can help with all these issues.

Some 30 percent of the population is missing the enzyme needed to convert folic acid (a form of vitamin B found in food and supplements) to 5-methyltetrahydrofolate (the form of B that our bodies can actually use). If you're in that 30 percent, you won't get as much benefit from the B vitamins you consume—*unless* you add 5-methyltetra-hydrofolate, better known as 5-methyl, when you ingest vitamin B. You have two options: You can get tested to find out whether you are missing that enzyme, so you know whether or not you have to take some 5-methyl whenever you take your vitamin B. Or you can simply finesse the question by always buying vitamins that include 5-methyl.

To support your hormonal health, you want to add nutrients to your diet that help with cell division and the body's ability to reproduce itself. Environmental stress, which we'll explore more fully in the next chapter, also adds to your body's burden, so supplementing with antioxidants can help restore health and hormonal balance.

To combat the effects of stress and restore hormonal balance, adaptogenic herbs can do wonders. The term *adaptogen* indicates that these marvelous herbs adapt to your body's needs. When levels of a particular hormone are too low, these herbs help raise them. When levels of a hormone are too high, the same herbs help lower them. I include suggestions for taking these herbs in the 28-day plan.

Finally, for hormonal and brain health, as well as for our overall health, we need essential fatty acids. We can't make fatty acids on our own, which is why we must make sure to include them in our diet. We need the right balance of both omega-6 and omega-3 types. Most of us get enough omega-6 in our regular diets, as this type of fat can be found in olive oil, eggs, meat, and poultry. Omega-3 can be found in flaxseed and fish, but I like to prescribe fish oil supplements to make absolutely sure you're getting enough. This supplement will help you have fabulous hair and skin, and it's also crucial for focus, energy, mood, and mental and emotional stamina.

WHAT WORKS: MOVE YOUR BOWELS ONCE OR TWICE A DAY

As we have seen, moving your bowels is extremely important both to move toxins out of your body and to promote healthy estrogen metabolism. Increasing fiber, drinking more water, and taking magnesium supplements can help, too. These are all elements of my 28-day plan, so if you follow that, you should see an improvement in your bowel function. If at the end of the month you're still not moving your bowels once or twice a day, please find a health-care practitioner who can help you resolve this issue.

Reconsidering Your Relationship to Food

As women, we are continually bombarded by unrealistic messages about our bodies. Almost all of us believe that we are too big, too small, too *something*. Almost all of us are obsessed, at least to some degree, with trying to achieve an impossible ideal of female beauty that even supermodels and movie stars cannot attain except by having their photos airbrushed.

So many of my patients have spent their entire adult lives on a diet! Like Chantelle, they are used to skipping meals in an attempt to lose weight and they find it extremely difficult to shift to a healthier pattern.

I'm hoping that by following my 28-day plan, you'll easily and gently learn what it feels like to eat the right amounts for your body, supporting your hormones while achieving a healthy weight. If you want to achieve a healthy weight, overcome insulin resistance, and balance your hormones, it is *crucial* that you consume the right balance of proteins, healthy fats, and fiber. If you find this difficult, however, I urge you to check out the Resources and get some help to make the shift.

I don't want you to overeat or binge on sugar, but I also don't want you to get through the day on a plain salad and a few slices of grilled chicken. Believe me, I've gone through this struggle myself, and I know how challenging it can be. But eating a balanced, healthy diet is probably the number one thing you can do for your hormones and your health. Please, do whatever it takes to make that possible for yourself.

WHAT WORKS: GET SUFFICIENT SLEEP

Sleep is vital for hormonal health and rebalancing, as well as for losing and maintaining weight. Sleep also affects leptin, which regulates feelings of fullness, and ghrelin, which regulates hunger. Furthermore, your body detoxifies while you are sleeping. As we've seen, your liver needs to be able to remove estrogen from your bloodstream or you'll end up with levels that are too high.

You also produce human growth hormone (HGH) when you sleep, which contributes to weight loss, general vitality, and overall hormonal balance. Since you tend to have less HGH as you grow older, sleep becomes correspondingly more important as you age. Generally, sleep is also crucial for balancing your sympathetic nervous system's "fight or flight" response with your parasympathetic nervous system's "rest and digest" response.

If you're having trouble sleeping, you might consider melatonin supplements. Melatonin is a natural hormone that helps set your sleep-wake cycle and your circadian rhythms. Over a 24-hour cycle, its levels rise in the dark—helping you to sleep—and fall when it gets light. You can increase melatonin through supplements but also through wearing a sleep mask, so that while you are sleeping your eyes are not exposed to even the tiniest bit of light.

Natural Sleep Aids

Try only one of these sleep aids each night—do *not* combine them. Do not take *any* of these sleep aids in combination with a prescription or over-the-counter sleep remedy unless you check with your practitioner beforehand.

- **Melatonin:** Start with .5 mg per night and work your way up to 3 mg as needed.

- **Phosphatitylserene:** 200 mg per night. This is a good supplement to take if you're wired at night, as it helps to decrease cortisol, helping you to switch from the stress response to the relaxation response.

- **GABA:** 500 mg taken with an apple and a few almonds—*do not take* without checking with your practitioner if you have low blood pressure, are on SSRIs, or are taking an MAO inhibitor.

- **Passionflower** and **valerian** teas can also help with sleep.

WHAT WORKS: GET MODERATE EXERCISE

The health benefits of exercise are so well known that I don't really need to repeat them here, except to say that exercise is terrific for maintaining hormonal balance, reducing cortisol levels, balancing insulin resistance, and building muscle. Exercise helps shift your body from sympathetic to parasympathetic mode, which helps with stress release, reduced cortisol, and overall hormonal balance. It also increases your levels of GABA and dopamine, two neurotransmitters that help you resist depression while boosting your energy levels and your ability to handle stress.

Numerous studies have shown that women who spend most of the day sitting have a lot more health problems than more active women. We don't yet know exactly why this is, but clearly our bodies were meant to move and react badly when they don't. Movement is also necessary for the function of the lymphatic system, which transports many toxins out of the body. Exercise also increases testosterone (great for your sex drive!) and human growth hormone levels (good for energy, weight loss, and overall hormonal balance).

I can't stress too strongly how important it is to find a type of movement that you *enjoy*. So many of us start out with great resolutions to exercise, only to give it up after a few weeks, just because life really is awfully busy and it's hard to find the time. I get it—but I don't want you to stop exercising. If you find something you love, you will make time for it, and then you get two benefits: the healthy advantages of exercise and the wonderful stress release of doing something you enjoy.

WHAT WORKS: QUIET, RESTORATIVE TIME

Remember that we always want to balance the sympathetic and parasympathetic nervous systems so our adrenals are supported and we aren't overproducing stress hormones. Each day, make sure you take at least a moment to quiet and center yourself. I urge you to do whatever you need to do to find that quiet, centered place—prayer, meditation, time spent in nature, or just a few minutes sitting by yourself—because reconnecting to yourself will make an enormous difference to your hormonal health.

WHAT WORKS: BIOIDENTICAL HORMONES

One of the greatest areas of confusion in women's health is the question of hormones and hormone replacement therapy (HRT). I personally do not prescribe the so-called synthetic hormones, such as Premarin, Prempro and Provera, but I'm a big believer in bioidentical hormones and may prescribe them when diet, lifestyle, and psychological support have not been enough to restore hormonal balance.

Unfortunately, the terminology here can be confusing because, in some sense, all hormones administered to women by health-care practitioners are synthetic, meaning manufactured outside the human body. The conventionally available estrogen (brand names include Premarin and Prempro) is a concentrated form of urine from pregnant mares. Conventionally available progestins (like Provera) are not quite the same as progesterone. There are subtle but powerful differences between these products and the hormones found in human physiology.

Bioidentical estrogens are also "synthetic" because they're made from plants in a lab. However, they are compounded to mimic much more closely the types of estrogens in the human body. In my opinion, bioidentical hormones do a better job of mimicking the two most powerful human estrogens, estradiol and estriol.

Bioidentical progesterone works in much the same way. Made from wild yams compounded into a cream, capsules, or various forms—troches, melts, gels, or drops—it mimics human physiology far better than the conventionally available progestins.

UNDERSTANDING HORMONE REPLACEMENT THERAPY

Historically there has been a great deal of controversy surrounding conventional hormone replacement therapy and I'd like to take this opportunity to clear some of that up. Back in 1985 when we first started Women to Women, we were considered renegades because we were *not* prescribing Premarin or Provera. At that time, HRT was the drug of choice for almost all practitioners. However, my colleagues and I weren't comfortable with this form of treatment, preferring to emphasize nutrition, lifestyle, and psychological support whenever possible.

Our position was seemingly validated by a 2001 study by the Women's Health Initiative, which indicated that HRT does *not* protect women from heart attack, stroke, blood clots, or the risk of breast cancer. Yet this study turned out to be flawed in significant ways. Most of the people in the study were over the age of 60. When they were suddenly given artificial hormones years after having gone into menopause, these older women reacted badly, showing increases in all kinds of medical problems.

On reanalyzing the data, they discovered that women in their 50s who had been given HRT after showing symptoms of menopause *did* derive major heart and bone benefits from the treatment with no increased risk of stroke or blood clots, and with a decreased risk of breast cancer. Although the 2001 study had been used to argue that hormone replacement therapy was dangerous for women, the problem was not with HRT itself but with the way it had been administered. You're likely to hear many confusing statements about hormone replacement, so let me talk you through the rest of the controversy.

First, you should be aware that HRT definitely helps protect bone and heart health. For example, one study showed that menopausal women whose estrogen levels were low faced a 21 times greater risk for heart disease than before menopause—making their postmenopausal risk equal to or even greater than that of a man. Replacing estrogen in some fashion would seem to be an important health goal for menopausal women. In addition, since the 2001 study that mistakenly offered a blanket criticism of HRT, delivery techniques for hormone replacement have vastly improved. Instead of being primarily available as an oral medication, hormones can now be taken as a patch, gel, cream, drop, troche, or melt. This alternate delivery system seems to decrease the risk of blood clots and stroke.

Meanwhile, no large, reliably interpreted long-term studies have been done on bioidentical hormones. At this point, we don't really know what the long-term effects are of either the commonly prescribed hormones or bioidentical hormones with regard to their role in promoting breast cancer. Some studies have shown that a slight risk—but only a slight risk—of breast cancer seemed to be associated with hormone replacement. But what we *don't* know—and what has never been looked at—is what happens when we prescribe hormones but *also* support the metabolism of estrogen down the healthier pathways in the liver. I personally feel most comfortable with this approach.

I can also tell you that the patients in my practice who get bioidentical hormones feel much better and show immediate relief of symptoms. This is what scientists call "anecdotal evidence"—not based on credible scientific research—but at this point, anecdotal evidence is all we have. Having said that, I'll share another of my opinions. I believe that the real danger to women lies not in the prescription of hormones of either type but rather in the estrogen metabolites that have been metabolized down the 4 or 16 pathways, as discussed in Chapter 3. I think that when we do have data, they will show that the most important protection comes not from avoiding hormone replacement but from encouraging estrogen to metabolize down the 2 pathway through diet and lifestyle as well as the appropriate supplements. In my opinion, when those steps are taken, it will probably prove to be safe to rely upon bioidentical hormones for some.

Accordingly, I prescribe bioidentical hormones, and twice each year I test my patients who take them. Once a year I prescribe a urine test for the presence of metabolites resulting from metabolism down the 2, 4, and 16 pathways because the presence of 4 metabolites—the most dangerous kind—can only be detected in the urine. And once a year I also prescribe a blood test to discover the levels of all the sex hormones and the 2 and 16 metabolites.

Generally, I want women to try my 28-day plan first and then, if that doesn't provide sufficient relief, to consider bioidentical hormones, rather than starting right off with hormone treatments. However, once my patients enter menopause, I have seen very few who did not need some form of estrogen administered vaginally. As we age, if the vagina does not receive hormonal support, it often becomes atrophic (wastes away) and loses its suppleness. Women often develop atrophic vaginitis, an inflammation of the vagina and thinning of the vaginal tissue, which can result in urinary incontinence and painful intercourse. In some cases the vagina loses some of its integrity, the clitoris becomes much smaller, and sexual function is compromised. If vaginal cream can prevent this, I'm all for it.

Whenever I prescribe estrogen, I always prescribe progesterone as well. This is crucial if my patient has a uterus because estrogen causes the uterine lining to thicken, and we need the opposing effects of progesterone to flush it out. Without progesterone, troublesome health problems might occur. But even for my patients who have had hysterectomies, I always prescribe estrogen and progesterone together because I'm keeping the hormonal symphony in mind. I want to be sure all the sex hormones are balanced, which means that I test for DHEA and testosterone as well. Often, I prescribe replacements for all four sex hormones, just to keep the symphony in balance. (For details on the kinds of bioidentical hormones that might be right for you, see the 28-day plan.)

What about HGH Supplementation?

I know many health experts swear by human growth hormone supplementation, a treatment widely popularized by Suzanne Somers. I have chosen not to prescribe HGH supplements, but I know many people who feel very strongly that these supplements have changed their lives. This is one of those areas where you'll need to review the facts yourself and then come to your own conclusions.

GIVE YOUR SYSTEM A BREAK!

In this chapter I've shared with you the basics of a hormone-health approach: diet, supplements, lifestyle, and, potentially, bioidentical hormones. All of this works best, however, when you remove as many burdens from your body as possible. In the next chapter we'll take a closer looks at ways to relieve your system of environmental and psychological stressors.

CHAPTER 6

GET RID OF THE HORMONAL DISRUPTERS!

I'm going to start off this chapter by telling you about Angela. Her story offers an amazing example of how our environment and the toxic burden it can place on the body contribute to hormonal imbalance. It also illustrates how the "body burden" of toxins and hormonal disrupters can be an unsuspected but powerful factor in our hormonal issues.

In Chapter 2, we saw that poor diet, lack of exercise, insufficient sleep, and psychological stress can burden our systems and disrupt our hormones. When we add environmental toxins to that burden, the strain on our body increases. Our stress hormones rise in response, setting off a hormonal cascade that can disrupt our insulin metabolism and many other aspects of our body, including our sex hormones.

Some of us may display greater resilience to this burden than others, revealing few if any symptoms. Even if we seem to handle our body burden easily, however, the added stress of environmental toxins might have subtle but powerful effects on our weight, appearance, mood, energy, and focus.

Some of us might be even more sensitive, displaying a significant response to what might seem like minor stressors. As we continue to pile new stressors onto the burden, we never know when the tipping point might come—when placing one additional burden onto our body suddenly results in major symptoms.

That's why I want you to realize the potential effects of environmental toxins and become aware of what you can do to clean up your environment. By eating organic food, drinking filtered water, using green cleaning products at home, and storing food in glass or ceramic rather than plastic, you can go a long way toward relieving the burden on your hormones, which will have enormous benefits for your weight, your hormones, and your overall health. Angela's story illustrates what a huge burden the environment can place on us—and what an enormous boost we can give our hormones and our health when we clean up our world.

ANGELA AND THE BODY BURDEN

Angela was a hair stylist in her early 30s who loved her job. She came to me with two types of symptoms: a premenstrual week marked by mood swings, cravings, and weight gain; and a mysterious skin rash that wouldn't seem to go away, persistent fatigue, and a tendency to catch just about every cold, flu, or virus that seemed to come along.

After running tests for various types of hormonal imbalance as well as other potential conditions, I found that Angela was indeed suffering from severe PMS caused by all the different types of hormonal imbalance we have been looking at so far, including an excess of cortisol and adrenaline caused by stress and an imbalance of insulin caused by her high-carb diet.

The second cluster of symptoms was slightly more difficult to diagnose because I had to run additional tests to rule out a number of possibilities. Eventually, though, I was able to identify the second group of symptoms as evidence of environmental sensitivity, probably set off by the various treatments Angela used at her salon. The chemicals in these products added to Angela's body burden, which already included a high-carb diet lacking in essential nutrients, insufficient exercise, troubled sleep, and emotional stress (Angela was coping with a learning-disabled child and a recent divorce). The rash, fatigue, and weakened resistance to infection all seemed to be signs that Angela's immune system had begun to falter under the combined weight of her *body burden:* the cumulative effect of all the stresses and strains in her life.

One crucial part of the body burden is the toxins, additives, and preservatives that we encounter continually in the food we eat, the water we drink, and the air we breathe.

However, the body burden is not only the result of environmental pollutants. All the factors we have considered throughout this book—stress, poor diet, lack of sleep and exercise—contribute to that burden. At some point, the cumulative effects of all these factors can get to be too much for a particular person. Symptoms such as Angela's rash, fatigue, and vulnerability to infection might well be the result.

Indeed, Angela's body burden seemed to be making her hormonal symptoms worse as well, for she had begun to experience premenstrual migraines, anxiety, and weight gain. I believed that she had reached a tipping point where both her immune system and her hormones were beginning to show increasing signs of stress.

The whole process reminded me of something that my colleague Mark Hyman, M.D., likes to say about functional medicine. He explains that functional medicine is a search for ways to right the imbalances in a few of the body's key systems. These imbalances might be caused by too much of something or not enough of something else. We might be suffering from too many toxins, microbes, or allergens, or from too much bad food and stress. At the same time, we might also be suffering from insufficient real whole food, nutrients, vitamins, minerals, light, water, air, or sleep; or perhaps from not enough movement, rhythm, love, connection, meaning, or purpose.

I tried to explain these concepts to Angela, and she nodded slowly.

"So what I hear you saying is that what's happening to me is coming from a lot of different places and that's what's making me sick," she said finally. "Part of it is the chemicals I use at work. But some of it is the food I'm eating, and some is the air I'm breathing. Plus my stress and lack of sleep and no exercise and all the rest of it. It's all combining to create these symptoms."

"That's right," I told her.

"But then why isn't everybody else sick, too?" Angela wanted to know. "The other people at my salon aren't even sick—not like I am."

"First of all," I told her, "we don't actually know how these chemicals are affecting your co-workers. They may have weight problems, hormonal symptoms, or other health issues that are the ultimate effect of one more weight added to their body burden, the same way it happened to you.

"But second, yes, everyone is individual. You may simply be more biochemically sensitive to these stresses than other people. We know that environmental toxins are problematic for everyone but there is a continuum of what their effects might be. You happen to fall on the 'sensitive' end of that continuum. Your co-workers might fall more toward the 'resilient' end.

"Third, the other choices you make in your life—your diet, exercise, sleep, and responses to stress—affect your total body burden. It's rarely just one thing that results in environmental sensitivity, but more like 'one last straw that breaks the camel's back.' Right now, a lot of things in your life are putting a strain on your system. Those chemicals at your salon were just the last straw."

Angela wanted to know if this meant that cleaning up her diet, modifying stress, and otherwise following my 28-day plan would make it safe for her to work at the salon again.

"I'm not sure," I told her. "Right now, it's as if you are sitting down upon four tacks: diet, lifestyle, stress, and environmental toxins. All four tacks are causing you pain. But if we got rid of three tacks and didn't remove the fourth, you would still feel pain. We probably need to remove all four tacks." (This concept of the tacks was first coined by the respected physician Sid Baker, M.D., and I have used it often since I first encountered it.)

"So there's a lot I have to change," Angela said finally.

"It won't necessarily be easy, but there is a lot that you can do," I reassured her. "Now that you have the awareness, you can take action. I'll help you take it step by step."

So Angela began taking one step after another as we worked to clean up as much of her environment as we could control and helped her detox to lighten her toxic burden.

First, Angela started drinking filtered water. She installed a water filter in her home and carried glass water bottles with her to work—glass, not plastic, so that she could avoid Bisphenol A (BPA), a contaminant in plastic water bottles.

Then Angela made some changes in her diet. She began to eat "organic only" as far as she could, although she made exceptions for Sunday dinner at her in-laws' house and for an occasional restaurant meal with her husband. "I want to keep it clean, but I don't want to get crazy about it," she told me. I thought she kept a terrific balance between cleaning up her diet and still being flexible when she needed to be. I also prescribed some nutrients to help her detox better as well as nutrients to help with estrogen metabolism, which eased her PMS symptoms.

Next, Angela began using only "green" products to clean her home. And just as she had stopped using plastic water bottles, she switched from plastic containers to glass and ceramic bowls to microwave and store her food.

Finally, Angela made the decision to leave her old salon and start up a new business by herself: one that used only "green" hair, skin, and beauty products, with none of the harmful chemicals that had created her symptoms. Because people were becoming more conscious of these issues, Angela soon had a thriving salon.

"I love being a hairdresser," Angela told me, "but I don't want to be sick. This feels like the best way."

BUILDING AWARENESS

Working with Angela reminded me once again how great an impact the environment can have upon our health—and how much we can do to make things better.

First, we can be aware that environmental toxins stress our system and overburden our adrenal glands, flooding our bodies with cortisol and other stress hormones that set off a hormonal cascade. As we shall see, there's a lot of evidence linking environmental toxins to insulin resistance and, in some cases, diabetes. Disruption of both adrenal hormones and insulin sets off a hormonal cascade that often affects the balance of our sex hormones as well. But once we know this, we can take steps to balance our hormones as well as to clean up our immediate environment.

Second, we can realize the extent to which these toxins block the effects of estrogen receptors (which is why we call them "endocrine disrupters") or even mimic the effects of estrogen (which is why we call them "xenoestrogens," or "foreign estrogens"). Again, we can respond to this challenge by taking extra steps to keep our hormones in balance by reducing stress, combating insulin resistance, and making sure we get the nutrients, herbs, supplements, sleep, and exercise we need, as well as by figuring out ways to modify and relieve stress.

Third, we can use my 28-day plan to protect our immune systems as well, since many experts believe that environmental toxins of all types are also disrupting our immune systems.

I've seen many patients with sensitivities that resembled Angela's, confirming my belief that the environment is a significant factor in addressing hormonal imbalance. Many toxins—in the environment, in home cleaning products, and in our personal-care products—have specific, problematic effects on our hormones. Fortunately, once you know how to avoid them, you can go a long way toward cleaning up your immediate environment and reducing your toxic burden.

I know it can be daunting to think about all environmental toxins in our world and it can seem even more daunting to find ways to avoid them. But I want you to be aware of these issues because I believe you can change things. You can change the products you use to clean your house. You can change the products you use to put on your hair and face and skin. You can change the food you put in your body and the water you drink to quench your thirst. You can change the way your liver detoxifies toxins and estrogens. And you can join with other concerned people and help clean up our world. All it takes is awareness and the will to change—in whatever small, personal way makes it easiest for you to get started.

ENDOCRINE DISRUPTERS AND XENOESTROGENS

Industrial chemicals, additives, and preservatives have two significant effects on our endocrine (hormonal) system. They either block hormones (and so are called "endocrine disrupters") or they mimic the effect of estrogen (and are dubbed "xenoestrogens").

Animal studies have suggested some dramatic links between environmental toxins and hormonal disruption. For example, adult male rats who were exposed to crude salmon oil developed insulin resistance and abdominal fat deposits. How much of our own obesity epidemic is the result of the environment?

Even more disturbing are the reports of African clawed frogs exposed to the common herbicide Atrazine (ATZ). Some 10 percent of the exposed males literally turned into female frogs who copulated with unexposed male frogs and produced viable eggs. This is a frightening image of hormonal imbalance caused by the environment.

The effects on humans are not nearly so dramatic, but we are certainly feeling the effects of environmental hormonal disruption as well. The literature is showing that the rate of childhood cancers is rising. In addition, we're seeing earlier puberty in girls and infertility among young men. For example, Danish research conducted in June 2002 found that 30 percent of 19-year-old men in the study had subfertile sperm counts—results that have been echoed in other international studies. And many experts believe that the childhood obesity epidemic in both sexes is at least partly fueled by the thousands of xenoestrogens making their way into our children's bodies.

Think of how many endocrine disrupters abound in our world: insecticides, fungicides, herbicides, industrial chemicals sold as detergents, resins, and plasticizers. In addition, the endocrine disrupters in plastics tend to leach out into our food when we microwave food in plastic containers or even when we store food in those containers. Likewise, the toxins from plastic water bottles leach into our water, further stressing our systems.

Once you start looking, endocrine disrupters seem to be everywhere. The chemicals used in most dry cleaning mimic the actions of hormones and are toxic to our livers, thus decreasing our ability to metabolize other toxins. Cosmetics and sunscreen are full of xenoestrogens, as are shampoos, conditioners, and body lotion. Toxins are found in the linings of cans, pesticides abound on nonorganic fruits and vegetables, and dioxins collect in the flesh of nonorganic animals. Baby bottles and nipples are often made of plastic, and when we run the bottle under hot water or heat it up inside the microwave, we cause it to leach toxins as well.

The problem is magnified because of our place in the food chain. As you move up the food chain, the concentration of toxins increases.

Recall the ways in which an industrial chemical might find its way into a plant. Perhaps it is sprayed onto the plant as an insecticide. Or maybe it enters the plant through the ground water that leaches through the soil. Perhaps it is an airborne particle that the plant absorbs by "breathing in."

Now suppose that an animal eats the affected plant. Most of the toxins in that plant accumulate in the animal's fat cells, where they remain more or less permanently. Over a lifetime of eating polluted plants, the animal accumulates more and more toxins.

If a meat-eating animal then eats the plant-eating animal, the meat-eater absorbs all those toxins, a process that is repeated each time the animal eats meat. We humans are meat eaters at the top of the food chain, so we continually accumulate toxins and store them in our fat cells. There, they stress our systems and potentially disrupt our estrogen-progesterone balance.

Prenatal Protection

A recent study discovered that some 287 chemicals could be found in the umbilical cord blood of newborns. When I learned this information, it became so obvious to me that we had an important issue to deal with. I felt the same way when I learned that the average mother has 150 chemicals in her breast milk.

Discovering these facts helped me understand that prenatal care was incredibly important, as was doing a detox before attempting to get pregnant. And by no means does this suggest that you should not breast-feed! Regardless of the body burden, breast-feeding is so beneficial to both mother and child that I would always encourage a mother to do so if that's what she wants.

If you're considering a pregnancy, work with a health-care practitioner who specializes in detoxification. Before getting pregnant, you can eliminate as many toxic chemicals from your system as possible, ensuring a healthier start for your future child. In the ideal world, you would allow a three-month break between your detox and your pregnancy.

ARE ENVIRONMENTAL TOXINS THROWING
YOUR INSULIN OUT OF BALANCE?

Fascinating new information has recently come to light about the connection between environmental toxins and insulin resistance. According to a 2007 study of insulin resistance in nondiabetic adults published in *Diabetes Care,* "These findings suggest that persistent organic pollutants (POPS) may be associated with Type 2 diabetes risk by increasing insulin resistance, and POPS may interact with obesity to increase the risk of Type 2 diabetes." A study in the *Annals of the New York Academy of Sciences* also linked POPS (a.k.a. pesticides) and other environmental toxins with insulin resistance.

Yet another study found a connection between environmental toxins and diabetes. People who are overweight and obese have generally been recognized as being at risk for diabetes. But now it turns out that the weight itself is not the issue—exposure to POPS is the key factor determining whether overweight or obese people will become diabetic. Those with a higher toxic burden were found to be at far higher risk than their less burdened but still overweight counterparts.

Obesity and insulin resistance have also been linked to the common herbicide known as Atrazine. Meanwhile, according to a 2008 study in the *Journal of the American Medical Association (JAMA),* diabetes has been connected with BPA. Another *JAMA* article linked BPA with "avoidable mortality" in the adult population.

These reports are just the tip of the iceberg of new research on the health impacts of toxicity, showing me just how big the problem is. What I know from the science and from my patients' stories is that we have a problem. It's up to you to decide what you're willing to do to decrease your body burden. The good news is that it's possible! My 28-day plan—including organic food and filtered water as much as possible—can begin to combat these environmental stressors.

DIOXINS AND DETOX

A number of hormonal conditions are associated with environmental toxins and xenoestrogens. Although no one knows exactly what causes fibroids, they are generally associated with increased estrogen levels. Some research suggests that fibroids may be at least partially the result of an inability to detoxify estrogens. If so, increased exposure to xenoestrogens would likely make the problem worse.

Likewise, in many studies, endometriosis has been associated with dioxins in the environment. As we have seen, endometriosis is a condition in which tissue from the uterus implants outside the womb: on the fallopian tubes, on the ovaries, or in the abdomen. Then the tissue sloughs off and bleeds with each cycle, bringing blood into places where it doesn't belong.

In theory, a woman's immune system should protect her from these effects. But as we saw with Angela, many young women are struggling with so much stress that the excess stress hormones partially compromise their immune systems. Indeed, some research is beginning to link endometriosis and autoimmunity.

My own personal speculation is that the tremendous stress that young women undergo puts their immune systems on hyperalert. Sometimes, some of the normal tissue from the uterus backwashes up the fallopian tubes, which we call *retrograde menstruation*. This can happen during a normal cycle, and the immune system should be strong enough to cope with the "intruder." But sometimes, weakened by stress, it is not. As a result, rather than being "zapped" by the immune system, the tissue implants and the disorder begins. Time will tell whether my theory is indeed part of this complicated puzzle.

Interestingly, I've never seen a woman suffering from endometriosis who was not also plagued with yeast overgrowth in her intestines. Often, women are suffering from gastrointestinal pain caused by the yeast, though they assume the pain is caused by the endometriosis. Finally, women with endometriosis tend to be estrogen dominant. I suggest that my patients with endometriosis avoid red meat and dairy products from conventionally farmed cows; these animals are typically treated with hormones, which tend to increase a woman's estrogen levels, further throwing off her estrogen-progesterone balance. Another solution is for them to eat organic as much as possible, since organically farmed cows are usually hormone-free. If you can't eat organic, at least eat grass-fed rather than corn-fed beef.

DETOX AND RESILIENCY

A few years ago, some legislators in my home state of Maine began to wonder about all the talk they'd been hearing regarding environmental toxins. They decided to conduct a study, which became known as "The Body Burden Study," in which they had themselves tested for heavy metals.

To their astonishment, they discovered that every single one of them had abnormally high levels of these toxic compounds. Even the 26-year-old woman who had initiated the study, young as she was, had accumulated quite a body burden already.

These results confirmed what I already knew: environmental toxins are a problem for virtually every single one of us. Now the question becomes not *if* I am affected but *how* I am affected, and to what degree. And what should I do to protect myself?

As I told Angela, individuals have a remarkably wide range of resiliency resulting from many factors: genetics, the particular place where we happen to live, the location where we spent our childhoods, diet, exercise, sleep, and stress. Our resiliency might also change over our lifetime, either improving as our health factors improve or weakening as our health factors worsen.

Just as we each have our individual resiliency, so do we have our own capacity to detoxify—literally, to rid our body of toxins. As we have seen, your liver is your primary detox organ. It acts as a filter, purifying your blood of substances that your body cannot absorb, including alcohol, medications, caffeine, sugar, additives, preservatives, and estrogen.

If toxins in the environment are flooding your body with xenoestrogens, your liver has extra work to do. This additional strain on your liver can have serious consequences for your health.

Even more disturbing is the way that toxins in your bloodstream are able to cross the "blood-brain barrier"—the barrier that keeps most ingredients in your blood out of your brain. Toxins, however, can break through that barrier, affecting brain function.

Moreover, these toxins tend to be stored in fat tissue. When people lose significant amounts of weight, they sometimes become sick as the toxins are released into their systems. Meanwhile, obesity means the body burden weighs even heavier as all those toxins remain within the fat tissue.

All of these factors work together in unique ways, with the result that in some individuals, just a tiny exposure to toxins can make a huge difference, while in others, even a significant exposure to toxins seems to have little effect. In all of us, however, the toxic burden of our environment threatens our hormonal balance. Fortunately, if we are mindful of this effect, we can take steps, as Angela did, to reduce our toxic burden while giving our hormones the support they need.

BEWARE OF GMOS

An additional environmental risk is the increasing number of "genetically modified organisms," or GMOs. Some 91 percent of the U.S. soy crop, 73 percent of U.S. corn, and 83 percent of canola has been modified, along with substantial portions of other fruits and vegetables.

Avoid the Toxic 12

One self-protective step you can take is to avoid the "Toxic 12," a list of the worst endocrine disrupters to be found in our shampoos, skin-care products, and cosmetics. Indeed, the list reads like the roster of most makeup ingredients! Read labels carefully and avoid products that contain the following ingredients:

- Benzoyl peroxide

- DEA (diethanolamine) and MEA (monoethanolamine) and TEA (triethanolamine)

- Dioxin

- DMDM hydantoin and imidazolidinyl urea

- Synthetic colors and pigments

- Parabens (methyl, butyl, ethyl, propyl)

- PEG (polyethylene glycol)

- Phthalates (xenoestrogens)

- Propylene glycol and butylene glycol

- Sodium lauryl sulfate and sodium laureth sulfate

- Sunscreen chemicals like avobenzone, benzophenone and PABA

- Triclosan

I find it significant that European beauty products leave out most if not all of these ingredients. For more information on where to find cleaner beauty products, see Resources or check out the website of the Environmental Working Group (www.ewg.org).

Genetic modification takes many forms. Soy and corn, for example, have been modified to withstand being sprayed with a powerful herbicide. Other crops are modified to produce their own pesticides. Although the manufacturers of these crops insist that these modifications are not dangerous to humans, it's hard not to wonder about their effects on our bodies. Some experts have claimed that the rising incidence of childhood allergies is related to these genetic alterations in our food.

Many scientists have warned against the risks of genetically modified crops but no one is completely certain of their effects. Since we don't know exactly how GMOs affect us, it probably behooves all of us to be more mindful.

However, the evidence against GMOs is gradually mounting. On September 22, 2012, for example, the results of a two-year French study were released, revealing that rats fed genetically engineered corn suffered from massive breast tumors, kidney and liver damage, and a host of other health problems. Female rats who ate the corn died at a rate that was twice or even three times greater than the control group (rats who ate food that had not been genetically modified). Male rats who ate the genetically modified corn developed tumors some 18 months earlier than their control group.

Another study, conducted over 10 years on rats, mice, pigs, and salmon, found that obesity was a frequent symptoms in those animals who were given genetically modified foods; it also found that they suffered from major changes in the liver, kidney, pancreas, and genitals.

In my opinion, these rather terrifying studies are yet another reason why we should consider supporting labeling laws such as they have in Europe. As informed consumers, we should have the right to know whether or not the food we eat has been genetically modified.

Avoid the Dirty Dozen and Choose the Clean 15

The Environmental Working Group (www.ewg.org) has put out a wonderful list called "The Dirty Dozen," which is the 12 fruits and vegetables that are most likely to be loaded with pesticides if grown conventionally. If you can't afford or would prefer not to "go organic" 100 percent, at least you can avoid The Dirty Dozen, making sure to buy those products organically grown or not at all. Since the list changes periodically and may well have changed between this writing and my publication date, visit the website to check out the latest Dirty Dozen.

The same website has a list called the "Clean 15," which lets you know about 15 fruits and vegetables that are generally safe to buy "nonorganic." So if, for whatever reason, you don't want to go 100 percent organic, you can use these lists to help guide your choices.

SPLENDA—NOT SO SPLENDID

Few of us are really aware of how many new Splenda products there are in the supermarkets. We've been told that this artificial sweetener is different from all the past failures—Sweet'N Low, NutraSweet, etc.—and that Splenda is the perfect sugar substitute: as sweet as sugar, but no calories; as sweet as sugar, but no surge in insulin; as sweet as sugar, but no side effects or long-term health damage.

The wave is coming because "low sugar" or "sugar free" is the latest fad—a welcome trend, given the health hazards of all the sugar in the average diet. But of the hundreds of new diet foods that will soon appear, most will use Splenda as a sugar substitute. This is important because for tens of millions of women, their diet soda or artificially sweetened food is a keystone of what they think are healthy nutrition and food choices—both for themselves and for their families.

On the other side of the argument are responsible experts who say that Splenda is unsafe—the latest in a succession of artificial sweeteners that claim at first to be healthy, only later to be proven to have numerous side effects. These authorities say that Splenda has more in common with DDT than with food.

What do I believe? I think that our regulatory system doesn't do a good enough job of ensuring our long-term safety. I'm concerned about the bigger picture, too: the dependence on sweets in the American diet to make us feel good—whether those sweets are satisfied by sugar or artificial sweeteners like Splenda. And I am especially sensitive to the women who can benefit from using artificial sweeteners as a bridge to a better life with healthier nutrition.

What should *you* think about artificial sweeteners? I want you to be fully informed about the dangers of Splenda (which isn't what food marketers want!) so you can make the best choices for yourself and for your family. So let's make sure you are.

I think of Splenda as a kind of public health experiment. Its popularity came along with the "low-sugar" craze, the natural successor to the "low-carb" craze, even though sugar and carbs are essentially the same thing once they have metabolized inside your body. According to the *New York Times,* some 11 percent of the food items on supermarket shelves will soon be labeled "reduced sugar"—most of those targeted at kids and their health-conscious moms. Sales in granulated sugar have dropped 4 percent. What's behind this trend? Splenda.

Products featuring Splenda are perceived as "natural" because even the FDA's press release about *sucralose,* the main ingredient in Splenda, parrots the claim that "it is made from sugar"—an assertion disputed by the Sugar Association, which is suing Splenda's manufacturer, McNeil Nutritionals.

The FDA has no definition for "natural" so please bear with me for a biochemistry moment: Sucralose is a synthetic compound stumbled upon in 1976 by scientists in Britain seeking a new pesticide formulation. It is true that the Splenda molecule is comprised of sucrose (sugar)—except that three of the hydroxyl groups in the molecule have been replaced by three chlorine atoms. I am not really crazy about the idea of you consuming chlorine, which is a potentially toxic substance and one that can function as an endocrine disrupter.

Indeed, while some industry experts claim the molecule is similar to table salt or sugar, other independent researchers say it has more in common with pesticides. That's because the bonds holding the carbon and chlorine atoms together are more characteristic of a chlorocarbon than a salt—and most pesticides are chlorocarbons.

The premise offered next is that just because something contains chlorine doesn't guarantee that it's toxic. And that is also true, but you and your family may prefer not to work as test subjects for the latest postmarket artificial sweetener experiment—however "unique." (See www.womentowomen.com for more information on toxins and persistent organic pollutants.)

Once it gets to the gut, sucralose goes largely unrecognized in the body as food; that's why it has no calories. The majority of people don't absorb a significant amount of Splenda in their small intestine—about 15 percent by some accounts.

So is Splenda safe? The truth is we just don't know yet. There are no long-term studies of the side effects of Splenda in humans. The manufacturer's own short-term studies showed that very high doses of sucralose (far beyond what would be expected in an ordinary diet) caused shrunken thymus glands, enlarged livers, and kidney disorders in rodents. (A more recent study also shows that Splenda significantly decreases beneficial gut flora.) But in this case, the FDA decided that because these studies weren't conducted on humans, they were not conclusive.

Of course, rats had been chosen for the testing specifically because they metabolize sucralose more like humans than any other animal used for testing. In other words, the FDA has tried to have it both ways: they accepted the manufacturer's studies on rats because the manufacturer had shown that rats and humans metabolize the sweetener in similar ways, but shrugged off the safety concerns on the grounds that rats and humans are different. In our view, determining that something is safe (or not) in laboratory rats isn't a definitive answer, as we've seen countless examples of foods and drugs that have proved dangerous to humans that were first found to be safe in laboratory rats, both in short- and long-term studies.

Here are two other reasons for my concern: first, in the 11 years since Splenda was put on the market, no independent studies of sucralose lasting more than six months have been done in humans. Second, none of the trials that were done were very large— the largest was 128 people studied for three months, making us wonder: what happens when you've used sucralose for a year, or two, or ten? Then there's the fact that Splenda, as a product, consists of more than just sucralose—it's made with dextrose and sometimes also with maltodextrin, neither of which were included in the original studies and trials of sucralose. So the reality is that we are the guinea pigs for Splenda.

And now, are our children the next trial group? Thanks to an agreement between McNeil Nutritionals (makers of Splenda) and PTO Today, which provides marketing and fund-raising aid to parents' associations, your elementary school's next bake sale may be sponsored by Splenda—complete with baked goods made with the product. By the way, the assumption is that sugar is the primary cause of the obesity epidemic. Believe me, this is only a piece of the story.

My advice? Stick with stevia, xylitol, and erythritol. They are healthier forms of noncaloric sweetener and very likely to be kinder to your hormones.

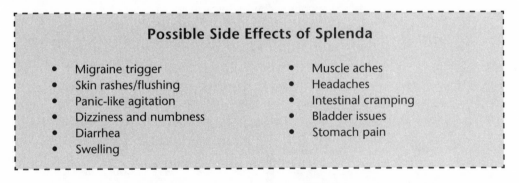

Possible Side Effects of Splenda

- Migraine trigger
- Skin rashes/flushing
- Panic-like agitation
- Dizziness and numbness
- Diarrhea
- Swelling

- Muscle aches
- Headaches
- Intestinal cramping
- Bladder issues
- Stomach pain

COPING WITH ENVIRONMENTAL STRESS

I know how disturbing this environmental information can be. Believe me, I've felt overwhelmed, too, especially when I've just done a workshop on the topic. But my intention here is not to alarm you or to stress you any further. Rather, it's to help you become aware of one more possible burden on your system and then help you find ways to lift

The Hormone-Friendly Home

- Focus on additive-free cosmetics and skin-care products. (See Resources.) This is especially important if you are concerned about estrogen dominance or are struggling with the symptoms of excess estrogen.

- Eat organic. If you're on a budget, remember that even Walmart has an organic section and that there are many low-cost alternatives online. (See Resources.) A local farmer's market might also be an economical alternative. If you can't afford to or choose not to go completely organic, remember the Toxic 12 and the Clean 15.

- Avoid processed foods and foods that are full of additives. Go through your pantry and clean out foods with multiple ingredients whose names you can't pronounce!

- Avoid genetically modified and irradiated foods.

- Use glass or ceramic containers in your microwave—and no plastic wrap on top!

- Use covered glass or ceramic dishes or bowls for storage—no plastic!

- If you must choose plastic storage containers, choose those marked #2, #4, or #5. When buying beverages, choose those in plastic marked #1.

- Use metal water bottles or those new plastic bottles that promise no BPA—no plastic!

- Buy canned food in BPA-free cans.

- When possible, buy acidic foods and beverages—including juices, tomato sauce, and carbonated drinks—in cartons, jars, or bottles rather than cans.

- Avoid toxic cleaning products and use "green" ones instead. (See Resources for some suggestions, or see www.womentowomen.com for homemade cleaning products that also work well.)

- Avoid synthetic fragrances and antibacterial ingredients in both household and personal-care products.

- Keep your home well ventilated and find ways to air out unpleasant odors rather than masking them with synthetic fragrances.

- See a biological dentist for an evaluation of your mercury fillings and/or have a heavy metal evaluation done.

- Work with a practitioner to use medical foods to help with liver detoxification.

- Work on improving your estrogen metabolism, as I explained on page 44. Consider getting your estrogen metabolites tested.

that burden. It's important to realize that you can take your own steps to change things in your own little way to make your body's burden lighter.

I personally would like to see our entire society decide to clean up our air, food, and water. Even smaller steps would be welcome. For example, the European equivalent of the Food and Drug Administration monitors cosmetics and skin-care products. Our own FDA ignores these products, however, so we're on our own.

Fortunately, we have an ever-increasing number of options these days for buying safer food, water, cleaning products, toiletries, and cosmetics. I've included a number of websites in the Resources section where you can obtain "green" cleaning products, cosmetics, and skin-care products. See the box on page 110 for some additional suggestions for creating a hormone-friendly home.

The other thing you can do is simply to be mindful that this might be a concern for you and your family. Then, if you suspect environmental sensitivity, you'll be prepared to take action. These issues affect each of us in different ways. Your individual vulnerability is affected by genetics, diet, exercise, sleep, age, and where you live, along with the cumulative effects of all the other stressors in your life. As a result, the xenoestrogens in your environment may have a minimal effect on your body or you may be affected more than you realize. The good news is that you can counter their effects by supporting your body through my 28-day plan, by eating organic, and by cleaning up your home environment. You can decide how far you want or need to go to avoid these environmental stressors.

CHAPTER 7

Sexy, Sensual, and Talking to Your Partner

Jennifer was a 27-year-old social worker whose job at a county agency involved working with people in extreme distress. She found housing for homeless women and their families, placed developmentally disabled adults in group homes, and organized support services for elderly people living alone. She loved her work but often found herself drained by the sad stories and difficult situations she encountered.

When Jennifer came to me, she was struggling with intense PMS symptoms that began two weeks before her period: menstrual migraines, fatigue, weepiness, irritability, and, as she put it, "feeling so jittery I want to jump right out of my skin!" She also told me that she and her live-in boyfriend hadn't had sex in three months.

"I'm always so exhausted!" she told me. "Half of the month I've got PMS, and I don't really like having sex *while* I'm having my period because it's so messy; that just leaves one week, and most of the time I'm not in the mood. Honestly, I didn't even realize so much time had gone by until my boyfriend exploded and said he was going to break up with me if we didn't figure this out. I can't really blame him, but I can't force myself to feel something that's not there, either. What can I do?"

Camille was a 36-year-old homemaker with two small children who worked part time at a local bakery. She came to see me about severe cramping during her periods, which she said had gotten worse over the last few months. Camille was also upset that she had gained weight after both pregnancies without losing it and was now about 20 pounds heavier.

Camille had struggled with postpartum depression after her second child was born, so her last practitioner had prescribed antidepressants. However, he had been unable to help her with the loss of libido that resulted. "I feel so deprived!" Camille told me. "My husband and I used to have a great sex life, and when things were so rushed and crazy, sex was our thing, you know? Even if we didn't have time for a movie, we always had time for that, and it was great! Not being able to enjoy it—I can't tell you how awful it is! And not even *wanting* it anymore—I don't even feel like myself. I know it's just a side effect of those pills, but it doesn't feel like a side effect—it feels like who I am now. This mother of two kids who doesn't even enjoy her husband—that's not me! Except it is . . ."

Isabella was a 45-year-old teacher who had never married. For the past ten years she had been living with a man whom she described as her "soul mate for life." She came to me for various symptoms related to perimenopause: weight gain, forgetfulness, loss of energy, mild depression, and occasional hot flashes. She also told me that she had basically lost all interest in sex.

"I'm not sure I was ever all that much of a sexual person," she said. "But now it's like I can't even *remember* what sex was like. I love Russell and I like living with him. But when we go to bed together I may just want him to hold me, and sometimes I don't even want that. He's so hurt, and he's being so patient."

When I asked Isabella what their sex life had been like before this, she shrugged.

"It was okay, I guess," she said. "Nothing special." And when I asked her if she and her partner had ever talked about their sex life, either before her perimenopause or now, she shook her head emphatically.

"Oh, no!" she said, "No. Talking to him about all of this? I'd be too embarrassed."

One of the saddest casualties of hormonal imbalance is sex. Women just don't feel sexy, sensual, or able to communicate with their partners when they're overwhelmed with cramping, depression, and out-of-control anger. The good news is that you *can* restore your sexual feelings and your sensuality. My 28-day plan can help you make a good start, and if that's not enough, bioidentical hormones can also help a lot. There are plenty of resources to help you reconnect to your sexual and your sensual self.

Communication with your partner can also make a huge difference. Men and women tend to communicate very differently, and what may be crucial is to understand the difference so you can communicate on his terms and help him understand yours. Alison Armstrong makes the excellent point that we can't expect our men to be like male girlfriends; that's simply not how most men relate.

It may take some work on your part to learn how to communicate with that understanding in mind. Finding a way to help your guy understand your hormonal challenges, showing him what works for you sexually, and finding out more about what he likes can be challenging. But doing so can all go a long way toward renewing your sex life and helping you reclaim your sensuality. (See Resources for information on relationship expert Alison Armstrong and her fabulous work helping men and women communicate with each other.)

BALANCE YOUR HORMONES—REAWAKEN YOUR SEXUALITY

I was concerned about the situations of Jennifer, Camille, and Isabella because I wanted them—and all my patients—to be able to enjoy sex. Yet so many women *don't* enjoy it. Here are some of the most common things I hear again and again from my patients:

- "You know, when my partner and I first got together, I was really interested in sex, but now that we've been together for a few years, our sex life is kind of humdrum. What's wrong with me?"

- "I've never really had much of a sex drive."

- "When people talk about how great sex is, I just don't get it. It's okay, I guess. But I can take it or leave it."

- "I used to have an amazing sex drive. But since I had my children and got older, and I gained all this weight, it just dried up."

- "My partner and I never have sex anymore. I don't really miss it and neither does he."

Sex is one of life's great pleasures, so what's going on here? In my experience, women don't enjoy sex for a number of physical and psychological reasons, many of which are interrelated. Here are some of the most common:

- Hormonal imbalance, including imbalances caused by pregnancy, childbirth, and perimenopause, especially low testosterone levels

- Too much emotional stress, which causes the body's resources to be diverted away from making sex hormones and into making stress hormones

- Overscheduling by either you or your partner or both, leaving little or no time for sex, romance, or intimacy

- Lack of sleep, a form of physical stress that also causes the body's resources to be diverted away from making sex hormones and into making stress hormones

- Insulin resistance, which contributes to imbalanced sex hormones

- Excess body fat, which contributes to imbalanced sex hormones and increased inflammation. Some women also feel ashamed of being overweight, which makes them feel less sexy and sensual because they don't like how they look or are worried about what their partners will think about how they look.

- Insufficient exercise, which contributes to a lack of testosterone, a key component of sex drive

- Poor nutrition, which causes nutrient deficiencies, which in turn can contribute to insulin resistance and/or hormonal imbalance

- Excess use of alcohol and/or recreational drugs, which can create hormonal imbalance

- Antidepressants, whose side effects include lowered libido

- Birth-control pills, whose side effects include lowered libido

- Other medications with a similar side effect, including blood pressure medications

- Growing up with negative attitudes toward sex

- Having a negative body image—feeling unattractive or ashamed of one's body

- Early unpleasant experiences with sex, including childhood sexual abuse

- Insensitive or unskilled partners

- A partner with a history of prostate cancer or who has had his prostate removed, who may have erectile dysfunction and therefore decreased desire

- A partner with erectile dysfunction related to obesity, diabetes, and/or cardiovascular disease

- Difficulty communicating with partners about sex or about other emotional issues

- Conflicts with partners, particularly unacknowledged conflicts

- Anxiety and/or depression about relationships or other aspects of life

- Living with a depressed partner or with a partner who is uninterested in sex

- An alcoholic partner, or if you yourself drink too much alcohol

- A long-term relationship with insufficient or no effort to reawaken sexual interest

Sex is such a wonderful part of life, it always breaks my heart when I hear from women who feel unable to enjoy it. So let's take a closer look at what goes wrong—and how to put it right.

HORMONES: NOT THE WHOLE STORY

So many of my patients assume that when they don't feel interested in sex, their hormones are to blame—and often hormones *are* a big part of the story. Sometimes, though, hormones are only part of the story, and sometimes they're not even part of the story at all. With or without hormonal imbalance, so many other factors are involved, including your brain, your life story, your family background, your culture, your self-image, and your self-esteem.

In many cases, your life circumstances can contribute to your feeling more or less sexy. Think of the young mother who has been taking care of kids all day long. She's got vomit all over her blouse, she's been changing poopy diapers all afternoon, and she's just prepared her third meal of the day. Dinner ends, and she does the dishes while her husband, who has been working overtime, goes out and mows the lawn. By the time they get to bed, her husband doesn't have the energy to romance his wife, but he's still interested in sex. And she feels like he's just one more person wanting one more thing and she just doesn't have anything left to give.

A lot of things could change that picture. Giving the woman additional testosterone might make a difference. But remember, adding one hormone at a time is often not the answer; it's the symphony that counts. This woman also might feel sexier if she had a free hour away from her kids, when she'd have a chance to take a relaxing bath, read a book, talk to a friend, or maybe just take a nap. Perhaps her sex drive would be reawakened if she and her husband did the dishes together, using that quiet after-dinner time to reconnect, chat about their day, and remember why they once loved each other enough to get married. Maybe if her husband did the dishes *for* her, she would find herself *really* turned on!

Because we're all multitasking so much these days, it's often hard to be *present*, paying attention to one another and to ourselves. Perhaps if she and her husband just slowed down and remembered how important it is to be in the moment, that might go a long way toward reawakening their intimacy and, ultimately, improving their sexual experience. Or perhaps she and her partner would benefit from learning to communicate differently about sex, so that she could ask for what she wants without embarrassment and he could better understand how to please her without anxiety.

Another key factor in sexual interest has to do with how long you and your partner have been together. A great deal of scientific research shows that when a couple first falls in love, they may experience up to 18 months of intense excitement, including sexual excitement. Then, if the couple stays together, the sexual heat mellows and deepens into a more profound feeling of love. If the couple wants to recapture some of the old thrill, they need to find new ways to excite themselves and each other. (See the box on page 120 for some suggestions on how to do this.)

Sometimes we do need to tweak a woman's hormone levels, and when a woman tells me about her low sex drive, I make sure to run tests on thyroid and sex hormones, as well as doing other comprehensive blood work to ensure that other abnormalities are not present. But a woman's libido is not just the product of biology. Her self-esteem, her hopes and dreams, her creativity, her relationship with her partner—all of these play an important role in her sexual feelings, as do her sense of religion and morality, her ideas about what a "good woman" should be like, and her connection to her sensuality.

I am often struck by our culture's split personality when it comes to sex and sexuality, particularly for women. On the one hand, we have so many puritanical attitudes, which can make it difficult to enjoy sex or revel in our sensuality. On the other hand, we are bombarded by sexualized images that sometimes border on pornography, images that sometimes make it seem as though sex is everywhere. Isn't it interesting that, seemingly out of nowhere, the erotic novel *Fifty Shades of Grey* suddenly became such a big hit? Despite our publicly puritanical culture, there sure seems to be a lot of interest in sex and sensuality going on behind the scenes!

In such an environment, figuring out your own personal version of sexuality and sensuality can be challenging, to say the least. Is there a lusty, wanton, sexy woman inside you? Or perhaps a demure, flirtatious, playful woman who enjoys her sexuality to the utmost? Do you have within you a sensuous woman whose way of dressing and walking makes clear how much pleasure she takes in her body? Getting in touch with these parts of yourself can open you to a whole new world.

Humans are the only species for which sexual desire and functioning are not necessarily linked to reproduction. Every other mammal has sex only when the female is in heat, and can reproduce as a result. Only we have sex just for fun—or to express love. We're the only species with a female orgasm not linked to reproduction. In fact, we're the only species in which females can have *multiple* orgasms!

We're also the only species that continues to have sex long after reproduction is no longer possible. Did you know that the incidence of sexually transmitted diseases in nursing homes is equal to that among teenagers? In fact, having sex in their 60s, 70s, and 80s is more enjoyable for many people, including women who no longer have to worry about becoming pregnant, who are no longer taking care of children at home, and who have perhaps finally come into their personal and professional power.

"At this age, I no longer care what people think about me," one of my patients told me recently. "It's taken me an entire lifetime to get here—but I am certainly enjoying it now!" That sense of "It's my life, and I'll live it as I please" also created for her a new sexual freedom, as well as a sense of being *in* her body rather than wondering what her body *looked like* to someone else. Feeling free and empowered and in touch with her body, this woman got into a new relationship in which she was able for the first time in her life to tell her partner what she wanted and to ask *him* what *he* wanted. "I can't *believe* how much better the sex is!" she told me. "And I'm sixty-four! I wish I'd known this earlier, but I sure am enjoying it now."

I find her attitude inspiring for all of us, at any age. Self-knowledge, empowerment, and a strong connection to our own bodies are the keys to sexuality and sensuality—along with hormonal balance.

BALANCING HORMONES FOR SEXUAL PLEASURE

In most cases, if you're not enjoying sex as much as you'd like, your hormonal issues can be addressed by following my 28-day plan, in some cases complemented by bioidentical hormones. Here are a few of my most common suggestions, including the remedies I suggested for Jennifer, Camille, and Isabella.

Natural Ways to Reawaken Your Sex Drive

Solo

- Take up a sensuous physical activity: dancing, yoga, massage

- Get enough sleep

- Get more exercise—find a way to use your body that makes you feel physically alive

- Take a ballroom dance class. Tango and other Latin dances are especially good for having sexy, sensual experiences that can help reawaken your womanly self. African dance can also be very sexually and sensually grounding.

- Meditate: being *present* can often enhance intimacy, connectedness, and sexual feelings

- Learn tantric breathing

- Get some sensual or sexy underwear that *you* like, and that you can wear all day under your business suit or sweat pants

- Tune in to your sexual fantasies and explore ways to pleasure yourself while you fantasize. If you don't have fantasies, experiment.

- Develop some new fantasies from erotic or romantic books or movies

- Visit a sex boutique, in person or online, and pick out a vibrator or another sex toy designed to give you a solo experience. Many websites can be a little daunting, or even seem pornographic, but three good ones are www.passion parties.com, www.goodvibes.com, and www.bermanandberman.com

With Your Partner

- Do something sensuous, challenging, or exciting together: take up dancing; go rock climbing together; travel to a new and exciting place; learn a language together

- Learn to give each other massages, including erotic massages

- Explore the joys of edible oils, which can be found in versions that smell good, taste good, and are good for you

- Find opportunities to see each other "in your power"—doing something you're really good at or really love to do

- Explore tantric breathing together—research shows that it can be incredibly helpful in increasing arousal

- Explore your sexual fantasies together

- Develop some new fantasies from sharing erotic or romantic books or movies

- Visit a sex boutique, in person or online, and pick out some sex toys

For women with really severe PMS, like Jennifer, I test for hormone levels and the possibility of other abnormalities. Often, I find low progesterone levels relative to estrogen levels. Frequently, helping estrogen metabolism by making dietary changes, increasing exercise, increasing sleep, and using nutrients to help liver detoxification can make a big difference.

I might also prescribe some progesterone cream to begin midcycle, around day 14, and to continue until the period begins. You can buy progesterone cream over the counter, but if symptoms are very severe, the OTC dosage may be too low to do you much good, so I would advise working with a medical practitioner.

If symptoms are very severe or if the progesterone cream hasn't helped, I might suggest micronized progesterone tablets in a time-release form. These, too, would be taken from about day 14 through the end of the cycle. You can also make the progesterone into a troche, a gummy bear–like preparation that would also be taken midcycle through the period.

Jennifer tried the progesterone cream and soon found relief from her PMS symptoms. She also went on my 28-day plan. Eating healthy food, getting good exercise, and enjoying restful sleep did a great deal to improve Jennifer's energy and mood—and her libido. Jennifer also committed to finding more "alone time" to restore herself, and more "couples time" to reconnect with her boyfriend. For all those reasons, her sex life gradually improved.

Camille's situation was a bit more complicated. To treat her postpartum depression as well as her libido, I wanted her to change her diet, do some exercise, get more rest, and find more time for herself. I encouraged her to find people who could sit with her kids for a few hours now and then so she could connect both to herself and her partner. I suggested that they commit to a weekly "date night" so they could rediscover each other again.

Because Camille was breast-feeding, I didn't want to recommend hormones, but I believed that the other elements of my 28-day plan would help her—and over time they did. She and her husband didn't find it easy to make time for themselves but when they did, they found that taking the time to breathe and be with each other allowed them to reconnect to their earlier passion. Having regular sex with her husband again was also good for Camille's physical and mental well-being.

For Isabella, I suggested a combination that I frequently prescribe for perimenopausal women: a combination of estriol, testosterone, and DHEA in a vaginal cream. This compound is unbelievable at helping to revitalize the vagina. It plumps up the vaginal walls, relieving vaginal pain, and it's also amazingly effective at increasing libido, which I find so powerful and exciting.

Isabella had excellent results with this preparation. She found physical relief from her symptoms, and she discovered a whole new world as well. The support for her hormones enabled her to experience a different relationship with her body, her sexuality, and her sensuality. At my suggestion, she and her partner signed up for a ballroom dancing class, and they used their time on the dance floor to discover a new kind of intimacy. Isabella also took some of my suggestions for speaking up more during sexual encounters with her partner, being clearer about what she liked and wanted. Isabella told me that she was starting to have sex more often and that she had begun to enjoy her body and her sensuality in a new way. She was looking forward to seeing what the future would bring.

PROTECT YOUR VAGINA

Many women develop bladder problems, particularly in perimenopause. Either they begin to notice frequent infections or they start urinating a little whenever they run, jump, laugh, or sneeze (this is known as *stress incontinence*). Some women also develop urge incontinence, where they suddenly need to urinate and find it very difficult to control their bladders long enough to reach a bathroom.

All of these symptoms can be helped through the use of a specially compounded estriol/testosterone/DHEA vaginal cream and with pelvic physical therapy. A pelvic physical therapist can help you use biofeedback to discover the power of your vaginal muscles, which can help a great deal with vaginal support.

Some women need even more vaginal support in the form of localized estrogen. Without it, they can literally lose much of the integrity of the vagina. So if you're someone who has a great deal of pain with intercourse caused by lack of estrogen, know that there are very easy and effective interventions available.

Another source of sexual pain can be endometriosis. As we've seen, endometriosis can be addressed through diet, exercise, and the other elements of the 28-day plan. In most cases, that's enough to relieve symptoms, but if sexual pain is severe, surgical intervention might be needed.

When it comes to sex, many women grin and bear it until they can't any more. But it doesn't have to be that way! Knowing that things can be different can help empower you to get the help you need so you can enjoy sex.

The Joys of Anatomy

If you have questions about your own sexual anatomy, including the role of the clitoris, the vagina, and the "g-spot" in achieving orgasm, I suggest you check out *Women's Bodies, Women's Wisdom,* by my former colleague Christiane Northrup, M.D. Chris does a terrific job of both talking you through the physical part of sex and exploring many of the issues that keep women from fully experiencing sexual pleasure. You can also go to my website, www.womentowomen.com.

SEX IS GOOD FOR YOUR HEALTH

I want you to enjoy sex because it's such a wonderful, exciting part of who we are. But as a health-care practitioner, I'd also like to let you know that sex is good for your health! According to Daniel Amen, M.D.'s book *Sex on the Brain,* there is an association between regular sex and regular menstrual cycles, lighter periods, better bladder control, fewer colds and fevers, reduced stress, less physical pain, and better weight control. Women who are having regular sex tend to stay in better shape—and they're usually in a better mood!

Last but not least, regular sex helps balance our hormones and neurotransmitters. This is a significant piece of the puzzle that many people are not aware of. Yes, sex is affected by your hormones but it also *affects* your hormones, so that women who have regular sex tend to have increased testosterone and estrogen levels.

NITRIC OXIDE: ANOTHER FEEL-GOOD BIOCHEMICAL

Another important mood booster and contributor to sexual health is *nitric oxide,* an odorless gas that works on the same principle as Viagra. Nitric oxide helps blood vessel walls relax so blood vessels open, improving circulation throughout the entire body. This is good for your heart, your lungs, and your brain. It decreases inflammation, which is associated with numerous health risks, and it's terrific for combating stress.

Nitric oxide supports white blood cells in their fight against infections and tumors. It also contributes to the decreased stickiness of blood vessels, which is terrific for cardiovascular health.

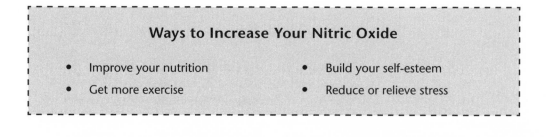

Ways to Increase Your Nitric Oxide

- Improve your nutrition
- Get more exercise
- Build your self-esteem
- Reduce or relieve stress

LEARNING TO LOVE OUR BODIES

I'll never forget it. I was sitting with my beautiful four-year-old daughter, getting ready to do a workshop for women on self-esteem. I had raised my daughter in what I hoped was a very loving and supportive way, trying to protect her from what I saw as our culture's damaging effects on women's self-image. A New-Age mom who had my daughter in a Waldorf play group, I was doing everything I could to give her what I saw as a healthy view of women's bodies and to insulate her from the culture's damaging views of women. I was so committed to keeping her away from problematic images that *Barney* and *Sesame Street* were the only television shows she was allowed to watch!

That afternoon, when I was giving my daughter a foot rub, I said, "Katya! You have the most gorgeous legs."

"No, Mummy!" my daughter replied. "My legs aren't thin like Barbie's!"

After I regained my composure hours later, I began to see that this was a much bigger issue than I had suspected. To my regret, I could not completely protect my daughter from the messages all of us get, from a very early age, about our bodies not being thin enough, pretty enough, *whatever* enough. So I used this as a learning and a teaching opportunity.

This culture is very, very hard on women. It expects every one of us to be the ultimate model of thin and perky and pretty and attractive, while a balding man with a big pot belly can still be viewed as attractive. I remember one well-publicized incident in which a fashion magazine airbrushed the thighs of a photograph of supermodel Cindy Crawford. When women's groups criticized the action, claiming that it was creating unreachable goals for women and their bodies, the editor said simply, "I'm trying to sell magazines!"

So many of my patients who come to me after a divorce or a breakup tell me, "I have to get in shape before I can even think of getting into a relationship!" They believe that no one else can find them attractive at their current weight or degree of fitness. Worse, they cannot find *themselves* attractive in that condition and feel shame at the very idea of being seen naked.

I contrast these women with some of the women in the Latin dance classes I've been taking recently. I watch women who are easily 30 or 40 pounds overweight sailing across the dance floor, shaking their hips in the most sensual way imaginable during a fast meringue number, or interlocked with a male partner, legs entwined during a slow, sensuous tango. As a health-care practitioner, I am concerned for those women and I'd like them to lose the extra weight that I know is not great for their health. As a woman, I admire them enormously. I wish all my patients could have that degree of self-love and sensuality—and I wish that for you, too! Our culture doesn't always make it easy, but the rewards are well worth it.

WHEN BONDING BECOMES BONDAGE

One key obstacle to women enjoying their sexuality is, paradoxically, their need to be loved. Many women get invested in a sexual relationship because they're seeking the love they didn't get as children or young adults. Sex releases powerful hormones, including *oxytocin* and *prolactin,* as well as the neurotransmitters known as *beta-endorphins.* All of these biochemicals have powerful bonding effects. Oxytocin and prolactin, which are also released during nursing and help the mother bond to her child, are higher while you have your period, which might help produce intense feelings of longing for a partner at that time.

So the sexual experience can bond you to people who may not necessarily be good for you but with whom you feel a deep, intimate connection that is driven by your hormones. Part psychological need, part hormonal response, these "bonded" relationships can be very difficult to escape, even when your conscious mind recognizes that the man in question is not right for you and may even be neglectful or abusive.

Significantly, we're more vulnerable to this effect when we're poorly nourished and/or hormonally imbalanced. When our beta-endorphins are too low, we crave sugar and white flour and we might be more likely to crave alcohol and drugs as well. The 28-day plan in the next section has a strong protective effect against this response, as do getting sufficient sleep and the right kind of exercise. Building your own self-esteem, finding what makes you happy, and believing in your right to the life you want can also make an enormous difference.

I suggest that my patients ask themselves the following questions to help define the boundaries of their sexual relationships:

- What works for you around the whole sexual experience?

- Do you know what you like?

- Do you masturbate and if not, why not? It doesn't mean that you have to, but I'd like you to at least ask the question.

- Are you comfortable asking your partner for what you'd like?

- Do you have a voice in the sexual part of this relationship?

- Are you comfortable setting boundaries—sexual and otherwise—in this relationship?

- Do you have regular orgasms? If not, begin to read and research why not.

- Do you enjoy sex? If not, have you ever?

If these issues are challenging for you, I encourage you to find a sex therapist, counselor, or support group whom you trust to help you work on them, and to consider some of the mind-body approaches I've suggested in the Resources section. Taking care of yourself sexually and emotionally can sometimes be challenging, but once again, the rewards can be well worth the effort.

TALKING TO YOUR PARTNER

To quote Dr. Amen again, your most important sex organ is your brain. What this tells me is that knowing what you want and then communicating it to your partner are a huge part of enjoying your sexuality.

To some extent, talking to your partner is a health necessity if you are having sex with someone new. I would also urge you to communicate about using a condom to protect yourself against STDs. Ideally, if only for health reasons, you would agree on safe sex practices. You owe it to yourself to have that conversation before you get into a new relationship.

Beyond the health issues, however, are the communication issues with any partner. Sex itself is a form of communication—one of the most profound and meaningful. Some of us have fantasies, however, that true soul mates, or at least good lovers, don't need to communicate in any other way. But communication is key to sexual pleasure in so many ways.

Having Safe Sex

Sexually transmitted diseases (STDs) are a fact of life, and new partners (or even old nonmonogamous partners) are a potential risk to your health. It's crucial to have a conversation with your new partner about his sexual history and yours, and for both of you to get tested. You want to test for herpes 1 and 2, HIV, syphilis, gonorrhea, human papillomavirus (HPV), chlamydia, and hepatitis C. Please remember that HIV tests might not turn positive for as long as six months after exposure. And until the tests come in negative, use condoms for your safety.

I know it's hard to talk to partners about these things but it's really important to do so if you're going to be sexually active. The conversation can be challenging but empowering—and lifesaving.

First, there is the ability of partners to help make each other happy. Whether you use words ("I like it when you touch me *here"*) or gestures (moving his hand to the part of your body you want touched or gently guiding him away from a touch you do not enjoy), communication can make your sex life better. This can be true at the beginning of a relationship when you are just getting to know each other, or later on when you are looking for ways to keep your sexual connection fresh and exciting.

Communication also helps set the stage for pleasurable sex. Maybe his beard is too scratchy for your sensitive areas and you need him to shave before you can enjoy intimacy. Perhaps he enjoys a particular perfume or a special outfit to get him in the mood. Letting each other know what you need is part of opening up to intimacy.

And then, ultimately, there is communication in the entire relationship. It's hard to feel sexy about a partner you're angry with or about whom you're repressing anger. It's hard to feel close to someone when you don't share anything intimate or important about your lives. For many women, opening up to someone requires trusting him in other ways, based on other kinds of communication.

One thing I've noticed is that women often communicate in words, whereas men are more likely to communicate through actions. A woman might tell her partner that she loves him or appreciates him, while a man believes that his actions—being faithful, contributing to the household, helping solve practical problems—demonstrate his love and appreciation. Learning how to appreciate each other's mode of communication can be an important part of developing trust, love, intimacy—and sexual closeness as well.

Talking to a Man

Some men aren't comfortable talking, particularly about sex. But a few simple questions can do wonders for your sexual communication:

- What turns you on?

- Would you like to know what turns me on?

- How can I make you happy?

- You know what would make me happy right now?

It's important that you have language to express your feelings inside and outside of the bedroom.

ALLOWING YOURSELF TO ENJOY SEX

If you came into my office and told me you weren't enjoying sex as much as you'd like, here is what I would tell you.

First, make sure you're eating a clean diet, getting moderate exercise and good sleep, and taking in all your basic nutrients. (Yes, you can find all of those elements in my 28-day plan!) If you're overweight, do what you need to in order to get your BMI (body mass index) into a normal range. (You'll probably lose weight if you follow my 28-day plan. For additional help with weight loss, there are lots of good resources, including my book *The Core Balance Diet*.)

Next, I'd get your hormones tested so we find out whether your hormonal symphony is in balance or whether it needs help from additional hormones.

After that I'd start talking with you about the nonhormonal piece of the puzzle that is always so important. I'd ask you how you'd rate your self-esteem on a scale from 1 to 10, and if your self-rating was too low, I'd suggest that you consider ways to feel better about yourself, including some of the mind-body modalities suggested in the Resources.

Then I'd ask you what kinds of relationships you involve yourself in. Do you choose relationships in which you don't feel heard? How sensual do you feel? How do you get in touch with your sensuality? What do you do for yourself on a regular basis? What do you need in order to connect with yourself? What can you turn to when everything is difficult or overwhelming and you need to let go of all the stress? Where do you find your joy?

I would help you explore the kinds of physical activity that can reconnect you to your vitality and sensuality. For me, it's dance, but for you it might be running, aikido, tai chi, or some other form of movement. What about pole-dancing classes at Mama Gena's School of Womanly Arts? (See Resources.) Does that sound like fun?

I would probably suggest that you find some wonderful new underwear that makes you feel sexy and sensual—for yourself, not necessarily for a partner.

And finally, I would suggest that you find out for yourself what it is that you need to do to inspire you to get in touch with the amazing human being that you are!

As this chapter concludes, I'd like to leave you with one simple message: sex is a wonderful part of life, so if you're not finding the sexual pleasure you deserve, I urge you to figure out a way to get it. You don't want to live the rest of your life without sexual pleasure! Why give up something that can be so much fun and can help you feel truly connected to another human being?

When I think of the wonders of sexual communication, I think of a couple on a dance floor, moving through the elegant, sensual dips and glides of an elaborate tango. He holds her, she curves around him, he steps back, she steps forward—the couple moves separately and yet together, savoring the music, the movement, each other. . . . When you see a couple engaged in an erotic, romantic tango, it's truly an amazing sight. Our lives should be like that—full of rhythm and passion, pleasure and connection. My hope for you is that you bring your hormones into balance, regain your health and the joy you take in life, and then dance the night away!

Part II

YOUR FOUR-WEEK PLAN FOR HORMONAL HEALTH

CHAPTER 8

THE PLAN BASICS

Here is your integrated step-by-step program to restore your hormonal health in four weeks, with complete instructions for diet, supplements, exercise, and sleep. If you follow this plan for the full 28 days, you will see significant improvements in your hormonal health. Maintaining this plan for three months should bring you dramatic improvement and relief from symptoms. Although it is not intended as a weight-loss plan, it will likely also help you lose weight.

This plan represents my "best practices" knowledge about what works to support hormonal health; achieve and maintain a healthy weight; and feel sexy, sensual, and energized for life. It is the way I have chosen to live, and in two and a half decades of practice, I've seen this approach work for thousands of patients.

However, I know that not everyone can make all of these changes right away. I want to support you in doing whatever you can, at whatever point you happen to be.

And remember, there are two ways to move forward from here. You can always go with Plan A, which I laid out on page 77. Or you can follow the specific food and lifestyle ideas that I list here and in the following chapters. While each week will have different elements, there are some "universals": guidelines that are good to follow no matter where you are in the 28-day plan or beyond. Here are those universals as they relate to diet, exercise, sleep, stress relief, and supplement guidelines.

DIET

- Follow the food plan starting in the next chapter.
- Stick to a regimen of three meals and two snacks per day (see Appendix A), so that you are eating about every three to four hours. Make sure to

have your first meal within 30 to 60 minutes of waking—the sooner, the better.

- Structure your meals so that half of your plate contains nonstarchy vegetables, one-quarter contains protein, and one-quarter contains high-fiber, low-glycemic carbohydrates.

- Increase your intake of cruciferous vegetables.

- Never eat a carbohydrate (grain, vegetable, or fruit) without also consuming some high-quality protein (lean meats and poultry, fish, nuts, seeds, or dairy products made from goat's milk or sheep's milk).

- Eat organic-only if possible, but at least avoid the Toxic 12 (see page 105).

- Avoid all sugar and artificial sweeteners.

- If you are still hungry at the end of a meal, you can have unlimited quantities of any nonstarchy vegetable.

EXERCISE

- Find a form of movement you enjoy, and engage in it for at least 20 minutes, three to four times a week. Possibilities include swimming, dancing, walking, biking, tennis, or yoga. You can also look on www.jjvirgin.com or www.slowburnfitness.com to find a "combination" workout. If you find something you love, you'll make it a lifelong practice, so keep looking until you find a way to move that really satisfies you.

- If you're challenged for time, see my suggestions on pages 63 for ways to work exercise into a busy day at home, with children, or at work.

SLEEP

- Get at least seven to nine hours of restful sleep each night.

- If you have trouble sleeping, follow my suggestions for sleep hygiene on page 62. Also, following are a number of supplements to help with sleep difficulties. Try only one of these sleep aids each night—do *not* combine them, and *do not* take *any* of these sleep aids in combination with a prescription or over-the-counter sleep remedy, unless you check first with your practitioner.

- Melatonin: Start with 0.5 mg per night and work your way up to 3 mg as needed.

- Phosphatitylserene: 200 mg per night. This is an amazing supplement to take if you're wired at night, as it decreases cortisol, helping you to switch from the stress response to the relaxation response.

- GABA: 500 mg taken with an apple and a few almonds—do not take without checking with your practitioner if you have low blood pressure, are on SSRIs, or are taking an MAO inhibitor.

- Passionflower and valerian teas can also help with sleep.

STRESS RELEASE

Build in 5 to 30 minutes each day and a half-hour to two-hour timespan each week to do something that relaxes you and gives you pleasure. Here are some ideas:

- A scented bath
- Time with a friend, in person or on the phone
- Time outdoors
- A quiet time with a good book
- Time to sing or dance by yourself or with others
- More play time
- Meditation or another form of spiritual connection
- A massage, from a professional, a friend, or a romantic partner
- Sex, cuddling, romance, or sensuality with someone you love
- More love connections

Try also to build in moments of peace throughout your day. Here are some ideas for that moment of respite:

- Go outdoors and stop to smell the air and feel the warmth or cool on your face.

- Focus your full attention on petting your dog or cat.

- Key in on a person you love—a romantic partner, friend, or family member— and allow yourself to feel the love that flows between the two of you.

- Create a fantasy—a sexual or romantic fantasy, or another type of fantasy that brings you pleasure.

For more comprehensive help with stress release, and to free yourself from historical stress, see my suggestions in Appendix D. If at the end of 28 days, your stress has not seemed to resolve itself, I suggest you have a functional medical practitioner check your cortisol levels.

SUPPLEMENTS

Following is a list of the supplements I recommend to bring your hormones back into balance. You'll see that I've recommended a high-quality pharmaceutical-grade multivitamin along with a number of other vitamins. I've done so because not all multivitamins include all the vitamins I would recommend—or they don't include them in high enough dosages. If the multivitamin you select does include the dosages of the other vitamins that I've recommended, you don't have to add the other vitamins as separate supplements. Just compare the ingredients label of the multivitamin you purchase with my recommendations and then figure out which other vitamins you might also need to buy.

Also, please note: I recommend that you increase your consumption of artichokes, pomegranates, watercress, and green tea. These foods promote general hormonal health, healthier estrogen metabolism, and optimal overall health.

If you are struggling with mood issues, anxiety, libido issues, cravings, PMS, painful periods, perimenopause, endometriosis, fibroids, PCOS, or adrenal problems, please refer to Appendix B for additional supplements to add into your program.

NOTE: These recommendations INCLUDE the supplements suggested on page 45 for healthier estrogen metabolism. Please do not double dose! Just take the supplements recommended here to support both your estrogen metabolism and your overall hormone health.

Breakfast:

- Probiotic with 20 billion mixed bacteria: one tablet before you eat
- A high-quality, pharmaceutical-grade multivitamin that includes 5-methyl tetrahydrofolate
- EPA/DHA-quality fish oil: 500 to 1000 mg
- I3C: one tablet
- Calcium d-glucarate: one tablet
- Flaxseed or chia seed: two tablespoons
- Soy: 40 to 60 mg
- Turmeric: 300 mg
- N-acetylcysteine: 600 mg
- Vitamin C: 1000 mg
- Resveratrol: 250 mg

Lunch:

- A high-quality, pharmaceutical-grade multivitamin that includes 5-methyl tetrahydrofolate
- Vitamin D: Have your levels tested and work with a practitioner to make sure they are optimal. Most people need to supplement with 1000 to 2000 IU per day

Dinner:

- A high-quality, pharmaceutical-grade multivitamin that includes 5-methyl tetrahydrofolate
- EPA/DHA-quality fish oil: 500 to 1000 mg
- Turmeric: 300 mg
- Red wine in the form of pinot noir or cabernet: six ounces if you desire
- N-acetylcysteine: 600 mg

Bedtime:

- Calcium: 800 to 1000 mg per day (bedtime)

- Magnesium: 400 to 500 mg per day (bedtime)

YOUR WEEKLY PLANS

In each of the chapters that follow, I lay out what a typical day would look like for you if you're living by my four-week plan. I also lay out a meal plan, and a shopping list that includes all the ingredients you'll need to make the suggested recipes.

CHAPTER 9

WEEK ONE

A DAY IN THE LIFE

6:30–7:00 A.M.: Wake up and lie in bed getting ready for your day. As you do so, take an extra five minutes to do the following breathing exercise. This type of breathing is extremely cleansing and relaxing. It's a great way to start the day because it sets your intention: to center on your own body and your own breath, present, alert, relaxed. Throughout the day, whenever you need a moment of peace, you can take one or two breaths and return to this state of calm.

> **Belly breathing:** Lying comfortably on your back with your eyes closed, place one hand lightly on your abdomen while you allow the other to rest loosely by your side. Through your nose, pull in your breath deeply, feeling your abdomen rise and expand as you breathe in. Through your mouth, lightly push your breath out, feeling your abdomen fall and contract down toward your spine. When you have gotten the feeling of breathing from your belly, breathe in on a count of two, hold for a count of two, breathe out for a count of two; breathe in on a count of four, hold for four, out for four. Continue on through six, eight, and ten; then breathe on a count of eight, then six, then four, then two. Take a moment to feel your entire body tingling with life as the breath continues to rise and fall in your lungs.

7:15: Drink two or three glasses of water or warm water with lemon.

7:30: Breakfast from the Meal Plan for the week.

8:00: Shower and dress.

8:30: Find a way to get in 15 minutes of brisk walking "as though you are late." You might walk to work; park farther away from work; or get out at a more distant train, bus, or subway stop than you normally do. Or, if you are taking care of children at home, put them in a "racing stroller" and walk briskly with them.

10:30: Have one of the snacks from the list on page 231 with a glass of water.

11:30: Make yourself a cup of green tea. Take two minutes to take ten deep, slow breaths, inhaling and savoring the scent of the tea.

12:20–1:00 P.M.: Take a brisk 15-minute walk. Then eat lunch from the day's Meal Plan.

3:00: Have one of the snacks from the list on page 231 with a glass of water.

4:30: Drink two or three glasses of water.

5:30: Once you are home, take another brisk 15-minute walk, or, if you prefer, ride your bike, rebound on a trampoline, dance in your living room, or find some other form of movement you enjoy. If you are ready, choose one of the workouts I recommend on page 134.

6:00: Make dinner from the Meal Plan.

6:30: Eat dinner from the Meal Plan.

7:00: Take 5 to 30 minutes for one of the forms of stress release I suggest. Even 1 minute is enough to get started!

7:05–7:30: Catch up with family, friends, chores, crafts, correspondence.

8:00: Read, journal, or meditate—begin to wind down.

9:00: Go to bed. Use the following visualization to help you relax thoroughly into a deep, restful sleep:

> **White Light:** Lie in a comfortable position with the lights out, ready to sleep. Begin to breathe deeply as you visualize a white light coming down to surround you. Feel the light entering the crown of your head, relaxing you as it

enters. Feel the light moving over your face, your throat, your chest, relaxing you and releasing your stress. Feel it moving over your stomach, your thighs, your calves, your feet and toes. Everywhere the light penetrates, feel peace and calm as you drift off to sleep.

MEAL PLAN

DAY 1

Breakfast
2 Homemade
Turkey Patties
1 cup mixed berries

Snack
Your choice—see
Appendix A

Lunch
Stuffed Zucchini
½ gluten-free roll

Snack
Your choice—see
Appendix A

Dinner
Rosemary Poached Chicken
Stir-Fried Chickpeas
1 cup steamed spinach

DAY 2

Breakfast
Crustless Asparagus Quiche
½ cup cubed melon

Snack
Your choice—see
Appendix A

Lunch
Herb-Crusted Salmon
Tomato Salad
½ sweet potato with
1 tablespoon butter,
sprinkled with cinnamon
if desired

Snack
Your choice—see
Appendix A

Dinner
Lemon Shrimp
Broiled Fennel
½ cup cooked brown rice

DAY 3

Breakfast
Berry Smoothie

Snack
Your choice—see
Appendix A

Lunch
Zinfandel Chicken
Favorite Broccoli
½ cup cooked brown rice

Snack
Your choice—see
Appendix A

Dinner
Pork Medallions
with Apple Relish
Slow-Roasted Tomatoes
½ gluten-free roll

DAY 4

Breakfast
Raspberry Avocado Smoothie

Snack
Your choice—see Appendix A

Lunch
Steamed White Fish
Green Beans with Almonds
½ gluten-free roll

Snack
Your choice—see Appendix A

Dinner
Lamb Burgers
Pecan Lentils
½ cup steamed vegetables

DAY 5

Breakfast
Protein Pancakes
½ cup mixed berries

Snack
Your choice—see Appendix A

Lunch
Leftover Pork Medallions
Leftover Slow-Roasted Tomatoes

Snack
Your choice—see Appendix A

Dinner
Saffron Chicken
Broiled Fennel
½ cup cooked brown rice

DAY 6

Breakfast
Easy Feta Scramble
½ cup cubed melon

Snack
Your choice—see Appendix A

Lunch
Eggless Egg Salad
½ cup mixed berries

Snack
Your choice—see Appendix A

Dinner
Turkey and
Vegetable Piccata
½ gluten-free roll

DAY 7

Breakfast
Eggs in a Nest
½ cup sliced strawberries

Snack
Your choice—see Appendix A

Lunch
Braised Tofu
½ cup cooked brown rice

Snack
Your choice—see Appendix A

Dinner
Spaghetti Squash Dinner
2 cups mixed greens with
2 tablespoons gluten-free dressing

SHOPPING LISTS FOR WEEK ONE

During the first week, there are two shopping lists—one to cover the specific recipes in the first week's meal plan and another to stock your pantry with ingredients you should always keep on hand. You can revisit this list each time you go shopping and simply replenish anything that has been used up during the week. You will also want to plan your snacks for the week and make sure to factor in groceries for those as well.

Week One List

Canned/Dried Goods

☐ 5 tablespoons (1 jar) capers

☐ One 14-ounce can chickpeas

☐ 1 can red kidney beans

☐ 2½ cups canned crushed tomatoes

☐ 1 small can diced tomatoes

☐ Two 8-ounce cans water chestnuts

Dairy/Dairy Alternatives

☐ ¾ cup unsweetened almond milk

☐ 19 eggs, organic if possible

☐ ⅓ cup feta cheese

☐ 1 cup goat, sheep, or feta cheese

☐ 6 ounces goat or sheep unsweetened yogurt

☐ 1½ cups plain unsweetened Greek yogurt

☐ 1 cup soy, rice, or almond milk

Fresh Produce

☐ 2 medium Macintosh apples

☐ 10 thin asparagus stalks

☐ ½ cup blueberries

- ☐ 2 heads broccoli
- ☐ 2 celery stalks
- ☐ 1 seedless cucumber
- ☐ 2 large fennel bulbs
- ☐ 2 cups mixed greens
- ☐ 8 lemons
- ☐ 2 limes
- ☐ 1 cup cubed melon
- ☐ 2 tablespoons fresh mint
- ☐ 1 cup mixed berries
- ☐ 3 teaspoons fresh oregano
- ☐ 2 tablespoons fresh parsley
- ☐ 3 red or orange bell peppers, plus 1 more red bell pepper
- ☐ 8 plum tomatoes
- ☐ 1 head romaine lettuce
- ☐ ½ teaspoon saffron
- ☐ 10 scallions
- ☐ 10 shallots
- ☐ 3 cups snow peas
- ☐ 1 spaghetti squash
- ☐ 8 ounces spinach
- ☐ 1 sweet potato
- ☐ 1 cup strawberries
- ☐ 4 medium tomatoes
- ☐ 4 large tomatoes
- ☐ 3 cups vegetables (your choice)
- ☐ 1 Vidalia onion
- ☐ 1 cup white mushrooms

- ☐ 3 cups sliced yellow summer squash
- ☐ 4 large zucchini

Meat/Main-Course Protein

- ☐ 8 boneless skinless chicken breast halves
- ☐ 1 pound ground lamb
- ☐ 1 pound pork loin
- ☐ 1 pound salmon
- ☐ 1 pound shrimp
- ☐ 2 packages firm tofu
- ☐ 1 package extra-firm tofu
- ☐ 1 pound turkey cutlets
- ☐ 3 pounds ground turkey

Miscellaneous

- ☐ 1 cup pecan pieces
- ☐ ½ cup white Zinfandel wine

Pantry Stocking List

Baking Goods

- ☐ butter
- ☐ cocoa powder
- ☐ cooking spray
- ☐ cornstarch
- ☐ ground flaxseed
- ☐ gluten-free flour
- ☐ gluten-free pancake and baking mix
- ☐ gluten-free vanilla extract

Breads/Grains

- ☐ gluten-free bread
- ☐ gluten-free bread crumbs
- ☐ brown rice
- ☐ gluten-free crackers
- ☐ steel-cut gluten-free oats
- ☐ lentils
- ☐ gluten-free rolls

Miscellaneous

- ☐ low-sodium, gluten-free organic chicken broth
- ☐ yellow onions
- ☐ gluten-free protein powder
- ☐ sunflower seeds
- ☐ 2 cans tomato paste
- ☐ 1 can diced tomatoes

Herbs/Spices

- ☐ basil
- ☐ bay leaves
- ☐ chili powder
- ☐ cinnamon
- ☐ cumin
- ☐ garlic, fresh or dried
- ☐ Italian seasoning
- ☐ marjoram
- ☐ mustard
- ☐ oregano
- ☐ parsley

- ☐ red pepper flakes
- ☐ rosemary
- ☐ thyme

Sweeteners

- ☐ organic honey
- ☐ molasses
- ☐ stevia

Vinegars/Oils/Dressings

- ☐ apple cider vinegar
- ☐ balsamic vinegar
- ☐ chili oil
- ☐ Dijon mustard
- ☐ gluten-free salad dressing
- ☐ hot sauce
- ☐ sugar-free ketchup
- ☐ extra-virgin olive oil
- ☐ oyster-flavored sauce
- ☐ pickle relish
- ☐ red wine
- ☐ red wine vinegar
- ☐ rice vinegar
- ☐ safflower oil
- ☐ sesame oil
- ☐ gluten-free soy sauce
- ☐ sunflower oil
- ☐ vermouth
- ☐ dry white wine

CHAPTER 10

WEEK TWO

A DAY IN THE LIFE

6:30–7:00 A.M.: Wake up and lie in bed preparing for your day. As you do so, take an extra five minutes to do the following exercise to cultivate gratitude. Gratitude is an incredibly healing and relaxing emotion, it is one of your best weapons against stress, and it is good for your hormones. Throughout the day, whenever you are feeling frayed, you can think back to this exercise to re-create the gratitude you felt.

> **Basket of blessings:** Lying comfortably in bed, visualize a beautiful empty basket. One by one, add blessings to the basket—things that you are grateful for: a person you love, a place you enjoy, even a body part such as an arm or leg. Keep going until you get to 20 blessings. Cultivating gratitude is one of the best stress releases there is—and excellent for your sex hormones.

7:15: Drink two or three glasses of water or warm water with lemon.

7:30: Breakfast from the Meal Plan for the week.

8:00: Shower and dress.

8:30: Find a way to get in 20 minutes of brisk walking "as though you are late." **Or** do a 20-minute workout from the choices on page 134.

10:30: Have one of the snacks from the list on page 231 with a glass of water.

11:30: Make yourself a cup of green tea. Take two minutes to take ten deep, slow breaths, inhaling and savoring the scent of the tea.

12:20–1:00 P.M.: Take a brisk 15-minute walk. Then eat lunch from the day's Meal Plan.

3:00: Have one of the snacks from the list on page 231 with a glass of water.

4:30: Drink two or three glasses of water.

5:30: Once you are home, if you haven't already worked out, you can do so now. Otherwise, take another brisk 15-minute walk or, if you prefer, ride your bike, rebound on a trampoline, dance in your living room, or find some other form of movement you enjoy. Your goal is to find a form of movement you love, because if you don't love it, you'll find it much more difficult to do and you're much more likely to stop.

6:00: Make dinner from the Meal Plan.

6:30: Eat dinner from the Meal Plan.

7:00: Take 5 to 30 minutes for one of the forms of stress release I suggest. However much time you were able to carve out last week, this week you might aim for five minutes more!

7:05–7:30: Catch up with family, friends, chores, crafts, correspondence.

8:00: Read, journal, or meditate—begin to wind down.

9:00: Go to bed. Use the meditation from Week 1 to help you relax thoroughly into a deep, restful sleep.

MEAL PLAN

DAY 8

Breakfast

Chia Breakfast Pudding
1 Homemade Turkey Patty

Snack

Your choice—see
Appendix A

Lunch

Leftover Spaghetti Squash
Dinner
1 cup sliced vegetables

Snack

Your choice—see
Appendix A

Dinner

Balsamic-Dressed Steak
Sautéed Escarole
½ cup cooked brown rice

DAY 9

Breakfast

Raspberry Avocado
Smoothie

Snack

Your choice—see
Appendix A

Lunch

Fast 'n' Easy Turkey and
Black Bean Soup
½ gluten-free roll

Snack

Your choice—see
Appendix A

Dinner

Steamed White Fish
Green Vegetable Trio
½ sweet potato with 1
tablespoon butter, sprinkled
with cinnamon if desired

DAY 10

Breakfast

Protein Pancakes
½ cup mixed berries

Snack

Your choice—see
Appendix A

Lunch

Leftover Balsamic-Dressed
Steak
Asparagus with Lime
½ gluten-free roll

Snack

Your choice—see
Appendix A

Dinner

Roasted Turkey Breast
Krunchy Kale
½ sweet potato with
1 tablespoon butter,
sprinkled with cinnamon
if desired

DAY 11

Breakfast
Melon Smoothie

Snack
Your choice—see
Appendix A

Lunch
Turkey Mango Salad
½ gluten-free roll

Snack
Your choice—see
Appendix A

Dinner
Bison Stew
Sautéed Escarole

DAY 12

Breakfast
Breakfast on the Go

Snack
Your choice—see
Appendix A

Lunch
Stewed Chicken
Warm Spinach Salad

Snack
Your choice—see
Appendix A

Dinner
Mexican Turkey Burgers
Pan-Grilled Portobello
Mushrooms

DAY 13

Breakfast
Don't Doubt It's
Delicious Smoothie

Snack
Your choice—see
Appendix A

Lunch
Leftover Bison Stew
2 cups mixed greens with
2 tablespoons gluten-free
dressing

Snack
Your choice—see
Appendix A

Dinner
Ginger Poached Chicken
Kicky Cauliflower
½ sweet potato with
1 tablespoon butter,
sprinkled with cinnamon
if desired

DAY 14

Breakfast
Salmon Roll-up
½ cup cubed melon

Snack
Your choice—see
Appendix A

Lunch
Leftover Mexican Turkey
Burger
Tomato Salad
½ cup berries

Snack
Your choice—see
Appendix A

Dinner
Quick and Easy Lamb Chops
Crunchy Broccoli Rabe
½ cup cooked brown rice

SHOPPING LIST

Canned/Dried Goods

☐ One 6-ounce jar marinated artichoke hearts

☐ One 14-ounce can black beans

☐ 3 teaspoons capers

☐ 2 tablespoons dried cranberries

☐ 2 pitted dates

☐ 1 cup refried beans

☐ 8 ounces organic tomato sauce

Dairy/Dairy Alternatives

☐ 2½ cups unsweetened almond milk

☐ 9 eggs, organic if possible

☐ 2 tablespoons goat cheese spread

☐ 2 ounces sharp soy, goat, or sheep cheese

☐ ½ cup soy, rice, or almond milk

Fresh Produce

☐ 12 cups arugula

☐ 1 bunch asparagus

☐ 2 avocados

☐ 2 cups broccoli florets

☐ 1 pound broccoli rabe

☐ ⅓ cup cantaloupe

☐ ½ head cauliflower

☐ 3 stalks celery

☐ 2 tablespoons fresh cilantro

- [ ] 1 small eggplant
- [ ] 1 head endive
- [ ] 4 heads escarole
- [ ] ½ cup fennel
- [ ] 32 cloves garlic
- [ ] 1 ginger root
- [ ] 21 Kalamata olives
- [ ] 1 jalapeño pepper
- [ ] ½ cup jicama slices
- [ ] 4 cups kale
- [ ] 5 lemons
- [ ] 4 limes
- [ ] 1½ mangos
- [ ] ½ cup cubed melon
- [ ] 1 cup mixed berries
- [ ] 12 ounces fresh or frozen okra
- [ ] 4 small yellow onions
- [ ] 2 oranges
- [ ] 4 large portobello mushrooms
- [ ] ½ cup radishes
- [ ] 1 cup raspberries
- [ ] 2 red onions
- [ ] 1 red pepper
- [ ] 7 sprigs fresh rosemary
- [ ] 14 scallions
- [ ] 6 shallots
- [ ] 12 ounces spinach or baby spinach

- ☐ 4 cups spinach
- ☐ 1 sweet potato
- ☐ 5 sprigs fresh thyme
- ☐ 4 large tomatoes
- ☐ 1 cup raw vegetables
- ☐ 1 Vidalia onion

Meat/Main-Course Protein

- ☐ 2 pounds bison
- ☐ 1 pound boneless top sirloin steak
- ☐ 2 ounces lean Canadian bacon
- ☐ 6 boneless skinless chicken breast halves
- ☐ 1 pound white fish (cod, haddock, tilapia)
- ☐ Four 1-inch-thick lean lamb loin chops
- ☐ 3 ounces smoked or fresh salmon
- ☐ 1 pound boneless top sirloin steak
- ☐ 3 pounds ground turkey breast
- ☐ 1 (approximately 2-pound) turkey breast half
- ☐ 8 ounces turkey
- ☐ ½ pound ground turkey *or* 1½ cups cooked shredded turkey

Miscellaneous

- ☐ 3 tablespoons sliced almonds
- ☐ ½ cup chia seeds
- ☐ 2 tablespoons flaxseed
- ☐ 1 cup chopped pecans
- ☐ 1 cup pine nuts
- ☐ 2 gluten-free tortillas

CHAPTER 11

WEEK THREE

A DAY IN THE LIFE

6:30–7:00 A.M.: Wake up and lie in bed preparing for your day. As you do so, take an extra five minutes to do the following exercise to cultivate gratitude. As I told you last week, gratitude is a powerfully healing and relaxing emotion and one of your best weapons against stress. That means it is good for your hormones, which is why I recommend going a little further with this exercise this week.

> **Basket of blessings:** While you are still lying in bed, visualize a beautiful empty basket. One by one, add blessings to the basket—things you are thankful for: people you enjoy, something that makes you smile, things you appreciate about your body. Last week you put 20 blessings in your basket. This week, keep going until you have 50 blessings. You can also appreciate that when you do this exercise, you are releasing stress and supporting your sex hormones.

7:15: Drink two or three glasses of water or warm water with lemon.

7:30: Breakfast from the Meal Plan for the week.

8:00: Shower and dress.

8:30: Either walk briskly for 15 minutes **or** do the 15-minute workout you have selected.

10:30: Have one of the snacks from the list on page 231 with a glass of water.

11:30: Make yourself a cup of green tea. Take two minutes to take ten deep, slow breaths, inhaling and savoring the scent of the tea.

12:20–1:00 P.M.: Take a brisk 15-minute walk. Then eat lunch from the day's Meal Plan.

3:00: Have one of the snacks from the list on page 231 with a glass of water.

4:30: Drink two or three glasses of water.

5:30: Either do the workout you have selected or do some type of movement that you love.

6:00: Make dinner from the Meal Plan.

6:30: Eat dinner from the Meal Plan.

7:00: Add a few more minutes to your time for pleasure and relaxation, selecting one of the activities from the list on page 135–136.

7:15: Catch up with family, friends, chores, crafts, correspondence. This week, consider going through your kitchen and replacing the plastic containers with ceramic, glass, or wood, which are healthier ways to store and microwave food.

8:00: Read, journal, or meditate—begin to wind down.

9:00: Go to bed. Use the meditation from Week 1 to help you relax thoroughly into a deep, restful sleep.

MEAL PLAN

DAY 15

Breakfast

2 Homemade Turkey Patties
1 cup fruit—mixed berries
or melon chunks

Snack

Your choice—see
Appendix A

Lunch

Buffalo Burgers
Tossed Greens with
Strawberries

Snack

Your choice—see
Appendix A

Dinner

Baked Chicken Breasts
White Beans and Kale

DAY 16

Breakfast

Spicy Veggie Smoothie

Snack

Your choice—see
Appendix A

Lunch

Turkey and Vegetable Piccata
1 cup mixed berries

Snack

Your choice—see
Appendix A

Dinner

Quinoa-Stuffed Peppers
½ gluten-free roll

DAY 17

Breakfast

Protein Pancakes
½ cup cubed cantaloupe

Snack

Your choice—see
Appendix A

Lunch

Super Speedy Shrimp Sauté
Cucumber and Watermelon
Salad

Snack

Your choice—see
Appendix A

Dinner

Buffalo Meat Loaf
Green Vegetable Trio
½ sweet potato with
1 tablespoon butter, sprinkled
with cinnamon if desired

DAY 18

Breakfast

Strawberry Cocoa
Smoothie

Snack

Your choice—see
Appendix A

Lunch

Quick and Delicious Chicken
Green Beans with Tomatoes
½ cup cooked brown rice

Snack

Your choice—see
Appendix A

Dinner

Quick Crab Casserole
2 cups mixed greens with
2 tablespoons gluten-free
dressing
½ gluten-free roll

DAY 19

Breakfast
Breakfast on the Go

Snack
Your choice—see
Appendix A

Lunch
Crunchy Salmon Salad
½ cup mixed berries

Snack
Your choice—see
Appendix A

Dinner
Steak with Parsley Sauce
Asparagus with Lime
½ sweet potato with
1 tablespoon butter, sprinkled
with cinnamon if desired

DAY 20

Breakfast
Super Spinach Smoothie

Snack
Your choice—see
Appendix A

Lunch
Easiest Beefiest Stir-Fry
1 cup cubed melon

Snack
Your choice—see
Appendix A

Dinner
Steamed White Fish
Green Beans with Tomatoes
½ cup cooked brown rice

DAY 21

Breakfast
Protein Powered Oatmeal
½ cup mixed berries

Snack
Your choice—see
Appendix A

Lunch
Cool and Creamy
Shrimp Salad
½ gluten-free roll

Snack
Your choice—see
Appendix A

Dinner
Spaghetti Squash Dinner
2 cups mixed greens with
2 tablespoons gluten-free
dressing

SHOPPING LIST

Canned/Dried Goods

- ☐ One 6-ounce jar marinated artichoke hearts
- ☐ 1 can cannellini beans
- ☐ 4 tablespoons capers
- ☐ 1 can chickpeas
- ☐ 4 tablespoons dried cranberries
- ☐ 2 tablespoons dates
- ☐ 2½ cups canned crushed tomatoes

Dairy/Dairy Alternatives

- ☐ 13 eggs, organic if possible
- ☐ 1 cup soy, almond, or rice milk
- ☐ 6 ounces sharp soy, goat, or sheep cheese
- ☐ ½ cup goat yogurt
- ☐ ¼ cup soy or goat yogurt
- ☐ 1 cup soy yogurt

Fresh Produce

- ☐ ½ apple, any variety
- ☐ ½ Granny Smith apple
- ☐ ¼ cup arugula
- ☐ 1 bunch asparagus
- ☐ 1 bunch basil
- ☐ 2½ cups mixed berries
- ☐ 1 cup mixed berries (or melon)
- ☐ ¾ cup blueberries

- ☐ ½ head broccoli
- ☐ 5 cups broccoli florets
- ☐ 1 Napa cabbage
- ☐ ½ cup cantaloupe
- ☐ 2 carrots
- ☐ ½ head cauliflower
- ☐ 8 stalks celery
- ☐ 1 bunch cilantro
- ☐ 1 large English cucumber
- ☐ 1 small English cucumber
- ☐ 1 teaspoon dill
- ☐ 1 head endive
- ☐ 3 bulbs garlic
- ☐ 1 ginger root
- ☐ 2 pounds green beans
- ☐ 10 cups mixed greens
- ☐ 8 cups kale
- ☐ 9 lemons
- ☐ 6 limes
- ☐ 1 melon
- ☐ 12 ounces okra
- ☐ 1 cup pitted green olives
- ☐ 7 onions, any variety
- ☐ 2 Vidalia onions
- ☐ 4 teaspoons oregano
- ☐ 1 cup parsley
- ☐ 1 peach

- [ ] 4 red bell peppers
- [ ] 1 yellow bell pepper
- [ ] 2 bell peppers, red or orange
- [ ] 1 tablespoon fresh rosemary
- [ ] 2 heads romaine lettuce
- [ ] 2 bunches scallions
- [ ] 2 shallots
- [ ] 1 spaghetti squash
- [ ] 2 cups organic baby spinach
- [ ] 24 ounces organic spinach
- [ ] 1 cup strawberries
- [ ] 3 cups summer squash
- [ ] 2 sweet potatoes
- [ ] 4 sprigs thyme
- [ ] 3 large tomatoes
- [ ] 11 plum tomatoes
- [ ] 1 cup tomatoes
- [ ] 1 large zucchini

Meat/Main-Course Protein

- [ ] 2 pounds lean ground buffalo
- [ ] 2 ounces lean Canadian bacon
- [ ] 12 boneless, skinless chicken breasts
- [ ] ½ pound crabmeat
- [ ] 1 pound white fish (cod, haddock, tilapia)
- [ ] Four 1-inch-thick lean lamb chops
- [ ] 1 cup cooked salmon (or one 7-ounce can)

- ☐ 1 pound salmon
- ☐ 2 pounds shrimp
- ☐ 1 pound London broil steak
- ☐ 1 pound sirloin or strip steak
- ☐ 1 pound turkey cutlets
- ☐ 2 pounds ground turkey
- ☐ 1 turkey breast half

Miscellaneous

- ☐ 3 tablespoons sliced almonds
- ☐ ¾ cup cashews
- ☐ 1½ cups pecans
- ☐ 1 cup quinoa
- ☐ 1 tablespoon tarragon
- ☐ 1 gluten-free tortilla

CHAPTER 12

Week Four

A DAY IN THE LIFE

6:30–7:00 A.M.: Wake up and lie in bed preparing for your day. As you do so, take an extra five minutes to do the following exercise to cultivate gratitude. This week you will again increase the number of blessings in your basket.

> **Basket of blessings:** Lying comfortably in bed, visualize a beautiful empty basket. One by one, add your blessings—think of everything you are grateful for, whether it is something big and important such as a loved one or something as little as knowing that you have your favorite herbal tea waiting for you in the cupboard. Last week you went to 50 blessings. This week, count up to 100.

7:15: Drink two or three glasses of water or warm water with lemon.

7:30: Breakfast from the Meal Plan for the week.

8:00: Shower and dress.

8:30: Either walk briskly for 15 minutes **or** do the 15-minute workout you have selected.

10:30: Have one of the snacks from the list on page 231 with a glass of water.

11:30: Make yourself a cup of green tea. Take two minutes to take ten deep, slow breaths, inhaling and savoring the scent of the tea.

12:20–1:00 P.M.: Take a brisk 15-minute walk. Then eat lunch from the day's Meal Plan.

3:00: Have one of the snacks from the list on page 231 with a glass of water.

4:30: Drink two or three glasses of water.

5:30: Either do the workout you have selected or do some type of movement that you love.

6:00: Make dinner from the Meal Plan.

6:30: Eat dinner from the Meal Plan.

7:00: Work your way up to a half hour of pleasure and relaxation, selecting one of the activities from the list on page 135–136.

7:30: Catch up with family, friends, chores, crafts, correspondence. This week, go through your kitchen and get rid of all the items that contain trans fats or hydrogenated fats.

8:00: Read, journal, or meditate—begin to wind down.

9:00: Go to bed. Use the meditation from Week 1 to help you relax thoroughly into a deep, restful sleep.

MEAL PLAN

DAY 22

Breakfast
2 Homemade Turkey Patties
1 cup mixed berries

Snack
Your choice—see
Appendix A

Lunch
Fast 'n' Easy Turkey and Black
Bean Soup
½ gluten-free roll

Snack
Your choice—see
Appendix A

Dinner
Ginger Poached Chicken
Stir-Fried Chickpeas
½ cup cooked brown rice

DAY 23

Breakfast
Salmon Roll-up
½ cup cubed melon

Snack
Your choice—see
Appendix A

Lunch
Orange Chicken Salad
½ cup mixed berries
½ gluten-free roll

Snack
Your choice—see
Appendix A

Dinner
Quick and Easy Lamb Chops
Kicky Cauliflower
½ sweet potato with
1 tablespoon butter,
sprinkled with cinnamon
if desired

DAY 24

Breakfast
Melon Smoothie

Snack
Your choice—see
Appendix A

Lunch
Oriental Tofu Stir-Fry
½ cup mixed berries

Snack
Your choice—see
Appendix A

Dinner
Roasted Turkey Breast
Krunchy Kale
½ sweet potato with
1 tablespoon butter, sprinkled
with cinnamon if desired

DAY 25

Breakfast
Eggs in a Nest
½ cup cubed melon

Snack
Your choice—see
Appendix A

Lunch
Warm Chicken Salad
½ gluten-free roll

Snack
Your choice—see
Appendix A

Dinner
Lemon Shrimp
½ cup cooked brown rice
1 cup steamed spinach

DAY 26

Breakfast
Don't Doubt It's Delicious
Smoothie

Snack
Your choice—see
Appendix A

Lunch
Turkey Mango Salad
½ gluten-free roll

Snack
Your choice—see
Appendix A

Dinner
Herb-Crusted Salmon
Pecan Lentils
Favorite Broccoli

DAY 27

Breakfast
Breakfast on the Go

Snack
Your choice—see
Appendix A

Lunch
Lamb Burgers
Leftover Pecan Lentils
½ cup mixed berries

Snack
Your choice—see
Appendix A

Dinner
Pork Medallions with Apple
Relish
Slow-Roasted Tomatoes
½ cup cooked brown rice

DAY 28

Breakfast
Protein Powered Oatmeal
½ cup mixed berries

Snack
Your choice—see
Appendix A

Lunch
Ginger Poached Chicken
Warm Spinach Salad
½ gluten-free roll

Snack
Your choice—see
Appendix A

Dinner
Steak with Parsley Sauce
Asparagus with Lime
½ sweet potato with
1 tablespoon butter, sprinkled
with cinnamon if desired

SHOPPING LIST

Canned/Dried Goods

- ☐ One 14-ounce can black beans
- ☐ 2 tablespoons dried cranberries
- ☐ 6 pitted dates

Dairy/Dairy Alternatives

- ☐ ¾ cup unsweetened almond milk
- ☐ 1½ cups unsweetened coconut milk
- ☐ 10 eggs, organic if possible
- ☐ ⅓ cup feta
- ☐ 2 tablespoons goat cheese

☐ 2 tablespoons goat cheese spread

☐ 8 ounces sharp goat, sheep, or soy cheese

☐ ½ cup soy, almond, or rice milk

☐ 1 cup plain nondairy Greek yogurt

Fresh Produce

☐ 3 medium McIntosh apples

☐ 6 cups arugula

☐ 1 bunch asparagus

☐ 2 avocados

☐ 4 ounces bean sprouts

☐ 3 cups mixed berries

☐ ½ head Chinese cabbage

☐ 1 head Napa cabbage

☐ ⅓ cup cantaloupe

☐ 2 stalks celery

☐ 1 seedless cucumber

☐ 1 head endive

☐ 1 ginger root

☐ 2 pounds green beans

☐ 2 green chilies

☐ 4 cups mixed greens

☐ ½ cup jicama

☐ 4 cups kale

☐ 4 lemons

☐ 4 limes

☐ ½ mango

- [ ] 1 melon
- [ ] 2 tablespoons mint
- [ ] 1 cup white mushrooms
- [ ] 2 red onions
- [ ] 2 yellow onions
- [ ] 1 orange
- [ ] 1 bunch parsley
- [ ] ½ cup radishes
- [ ] 2 sprigs rosemary
- [ ] 14 scallions
- [ ] 8 shallots
- [ ] 5 cups spinach
- [ ] 1½ cups organic baby spinach
- [ ] 1 tablespoon tarragon
- [ ] 2 sweet potatoes
- [ ] 1 large tomato
- [ ] 4 plum tomatoes

Meat/Main-Course Protein

- [ ] 2 ounces lean Canadian bacon
- [ ] 6 boneless skinless chicken breasts
- [ ] 1 pound ground lamb
- [ ] 1 pound pork loin
- [ ] 1 pound salmon
- [ ] 3 ounces salmon, fresh or smoked
- [ ] 2 pounds top sirloin steak
- [ ] 8 ounces firm tofu
- [ ] 1 turkey breast half

- ☐ 1½ pounds ground turkey
- ☐ 8 ounces turkey, cooked, cubed

Miscellaneous

- ☐ 1 cup sliced almonds
- ☐ 4 tablespoons cashew butter
- ☐ ¾ cup cashews
- ☐ ½ cup pecans
- ☐ 1 cup pine nuts
- ☐ 2 gluten-free tortillas

CHAPTER 13

THE RECIPES

Note to readers: Please make sure you wash all the fresh fruits and vegetables that you use, either with plain water or with one of the vegetable washes in the Resources section.

ASPARAGUS WITH LIME

1 tablespoon olive oil
2 cloves garlic, minced
1 medium shallot, sliced into thin rings
1 bunch fresh asparagus, trimmed, with tough ends removed
Juice of ½ lime
Salt and pepper to taste

In a large skillet, heat olive oil over medium heat. Add garlic and shallot, and cook for 3 minutes, stirring frequently. Add asparagus and stir gently. Cook until asparagus is bright green and has reached the desired tenderness.

Remove from heat and drizzle with lime juice. Season with salt and pepper.

2 servings

BAKED CHICKEN BREASTS

4 boneless skinless chicken breasts
1 teaspoon olive oil
Salt and pepper to taste

Preheat oven to 350 degrees.

Brush chicken breasts lightly with olive oil, season with salt and pepper, and place in a small baking pan.

Place in oven and cook for 18 to 20 minutes or until juice runs clear.

4 servings

BALSAMIC-DRESSED STEAK

6 cups arugula

2 tablespoons pine nuts, toasted if desired

1 pound boneless top sirloin steak, cut into thin strips

Salt and pepper to taste

¼ cup olive oil

3 cloves garlic, minced

2 sprigs fresh rosemary

2 shallots, thinly sliced

2 tablespoons balsamic vinegar

3 tablespoons red wine vinegar

Place arugula and pine nuts on a large platter.

Place steak slices on a baking sheet, then salt and pepper to taste.

In a heavy large skillet, heat oil over medium-high heat. Add garlic and rosemary and stir frequently until garlic is lightly browned. Remove garlic and rosemary, but leave oil in skillet.

Keeping heat on medium-high, add meat to skillet. Turn frequently, browning sides evenly until meat reaches desired doneness. Remove steak from skillet and arrange on arugula.

Lower heat under skillet to medium. Add shallot and vinegars. Bring mixture to a simmer and continue to cook for 3 minutes.

Pour dressing over steak and arugula, and serve immediately.

4 servings

BERRY SMOOTHIE

½ cup strawberries

½ cup blueberries

2 tablespoons ground flaxseed

6 ounces unsweetened goat or sheep yogurt

¾ cup unsweetened almond milk

1 scoop gluten-free protein powder

½ cup ice cubes

Place all ingredients in a blender and blend until smooth.

1 serving

BISON STEW

2 tablespoons olive oil, divided

2 pounds bison, trimmed of fat and cut into cubes

2 yellow onions, minced

1 small eggplant, seeded and cut into cubes

3 stalks celery, chopped

3 cloves garlic, minced

2 tablespoons gluten-free flour

4 cups low-sodium, gluten-free organic chicken broth

1 cup water

Salt and pepper to taste

8 ounces organic tomato sauce

1 teaspoon dried thyme

2 bay leaves

Heat 1 tablespoon olive oil in a large, heavy saucepan over medium-high heat. Brown the bison cubes in oil. Remove bison and set aside.

Add remaining olive oil to pan and add onions, eggplant, and celery. Stir frequently until softened. Add garlic and cook until lightly browned. Slowly add flour and mix well. Stir in broth, water, salt and pepper, tomato sauce, and thyme. Add bay leaves and bring to a boil.

Return bison to the mixture and stir. Reduce heat to low, cover, and cook until meat is very tender, about 1 hour.

Remove bay leaves and serve.

4 servings

BRAISED TOFU

2 packages firm tofu

3 tablespoons sesame oil, divided

Two 8-ounce cans water chestnuts

3 cups snow peas, trimmed

3 red or orange bell peppers, cut into thin slices

1½ teaspoons oyster-flavored sauce

2½ cups water

Slice each package of tofu into four slabs. Place each slab between paper towels and press out excess water.

Heat half the sesame oil in a large skillet over medium heat. Add tofu and sauté for 4 to 6 minutes on each side, or until lightly browned.

Remove tofu from skillet, cut into cubes, and set aside.

Add remaining sesame oil to the skillet. Add water chestnuts, peas, and peppers and cook until desired tenderness is reached.

Meanwhile, in a small bowl, mix together oyster sauce and water.

Add tofu and oyster-sauce mixture to vegetables. Cover and cook over low heat for 8 to 12 minutes, or until vegetables have reached desired doneness.

4 servings

BREAKFAST ON THE GO

1 gluten-free tortilla

2 ounces sharp soy, goat, or sheep cheese, shredded

2 hard-boiled eggs, sliced

2 ounces lean Canadian bacon, chopped

Lay tortilla flat. Layer cheese, egg, and bacon on tortilla.

Starting at one end, roll tortilla tightly around filling twice. Fold ends in toward the center and continue rolling until complete.

1 serving

BROILED FENNEL

1 tablespoon olive oil, divided

1 large fennel bulb, trimmed and cut into thin slices

Salt and pepper to taste

Juice of 1 lime

2 tablespoons grated goat cheese

Preheat broiler.

Lightly coat a baking sheet with half of the olive oil. Place fennel slices on sheet. Drizzle the slices with remaining olive oil and season with salt and pepper to taste. Drizzle half of the lime juice over the fennel pieces. Broil for five minutes.

Remove baking sheet from oven. Turn fennel slices over and top with cheese. Return to broiler until cheese melts.

Drizzle with remaining lime juice just before serving.

1 serving

BUFFALO BURGERS

½ tablespoon olive oil

1 cup finely chopped onion

1 clove garlic, minced

1 pound lean ground buffalo

1 teaspoon minced thyme

Salt and pepper to taste

1 egg, beaten

Cooking spray

⅓ cup vermouth

Warm oil in large skillet over medium heat. Add onion and garlic, and sauté until translucent.

In a large bowl, combine sautéed onion and garlic, meat, thyme, salt and pepper, and egg. Mix well.

Form mixture into 4 patties of equal size.

Spray a large skillet with cooking spray and heat over medium-high heat. Add patties and cook for 4 minutes. Reduce heat to medium and flip patties, cooking for an additional 1 to 2 minutes or until meat reaches desired doneness.

Add vermouth, cover, and cook for an additional 2 minutes.

4 servings

BUFFALO MEAT LOAF

½ teaspoon olive oil
½ cup gluten-free bread crumbs
1 pound ground buffalo
½ large Vidalia onion, minced
1 egg, beaten
1 ½ teaspoons dried mustard
1 cup diced canned tomatoes, drained
Salt and pepper to taste
½ cup sugar-free ketchup

Preheat oven to 350 degrees.

Lightly coat a loaf pan with olive oil.

In a large bowl, combine bread crumbs, buffalo, and onion.

In a medium bowl, combine egg, mustard, tomatoes, and salt and pepper.

Pour egg mixture into buffalo mixture and mix very well. Form mixture into a loaf and place in prepared pan. Spread ketchup over top and sides.

Cook for approximately 90 minutes or until desired doneness.

4 servings

CHIA BREAKFAST PUDDING

½ cup chia seeds

1 cup almond milk

¼ teaspoon gluten-free vanilla extract

Cinnamon to taste

¼ to ½ cup fresh berries, optional

Place chia seeds in a medium bowl. Add almond milk and vanilla, and mix well. Let mixture sit for 30 to 60 minutes, stirring frequently until chia seeds have plumped and mixture has a puddinglike texture. Sprinkle with cinnamon. Add berries if desired.

1 serving

COOL AND CREAMY SHRIMP SALAD

1½ teaspoons finely chopped fresh dill

½ cup goat yogurt

½ cup white wine

3 cups mixed melon, honeydew and cantaloupe

1 pound shrimp, chopped

8 large romaine leaves, chopped

Juice of 2 lemons

In a large bowl, combine dill, yogurt, and wine. Mix well. Add melon and shrimp; mix again. Cover and refrigerate for several hours.

Serve on chopped romaine leaves, and drizzle with lemon juice.

4 servings

CRUNCHY BROCCOLI RABE

1 tablespoon chopped pecans
1 pound broccoli rabe, trimmed and thick stems removed
1 tablespoon olive oil
1 clove garlic, minced
½ teaspoon red pepper flakes
5 large Kalamata olives, halved
Juice of ½ lemon

Toast pecans in a toaster oven or in a dry skillet over medium heat until golden brown. Set aside.

Steam broccoli rabe for 3 minutes. Meanwhile, prepare a large bowl of iced water. When broccoli rabe has finished steaming, immediately place in iced water.

Heat olive oil in a large skillet over medium heat. Add garlic and sauté until garlic turns golden brown. Add drained broccoli rabe, red pepper flakes, and olives. Cook until broccoli rabe reaches desired tenderness.

Remove from heat and add pecans and lemon juice.

Toss well and serve.

2 servings

CRUNCHY SALMON SALAD

1 cup cooked salmon (or one 7-ounce can), flaked
1 hard-boiled egg, chopped
1 small English cucumber, peeled and chopped
½ red bell pepper, seeded and chopped
¼ cup unsweetened soy or goat yogurt
Juice of ½ lemon (or more to taste)
Salt and pepper to taste
2 cups mixed greens

In a medium bowl, combine salmon and egg.

In a large bowl, combine cucumber, pepper, and yogurt. Mix well.

Add salmon mixture to yogurt mixture, then add lemon juice and season with salt and pepper. Mix well.

Serve on a bed of greens.

2 servings

CRUSTLESS ASPARAGUS QUICHE

6 large eggs

⅓ cup unsweetened soy or almond milk

1½ tablespoons chopped shallots

½ cup sharp goat or sheep cheese, shredded

1 teaspoon prepared Dijon mustard

Salt and pepper to taste

10 thin asparagus stalks

Juice of ½ lemon

½ teaspoon olive oil

1 medium tomato, thinly sliced

Preheat oven to 400 degrees.

Line a 9-inch-square pan with parchment paper cut to fit.

Break eggs into a large bowl and beat. Add milk, shallots, cheese, mustard, and salt and pepper. Carefully pour mixture into parchment paper–lined pan. Place in oven and bake for 10 minutes.

While egg mixture is baking, cut asparagus stalks to less than 9 inches.

Place lemon juice and olive oil in a large bowl. Add asparagus stalks and toss well.

Remove egg mixture from oven and place asparagus stalks neatly in a row on top of egg mixture. Place tomato slices on top of asparagus, and return to oven and cook for another 10 to 15 minutes or until center is set.

Remove from oven and let cool for 10 minutes.

Loosening parchment paper, carefully remove quiche from baking dish.

2 servings

CUCUMBER AND WATERMELON SALAD

1 large English cucumber, peeled and cubed
2 cups seedless watermelon, cubed
Juice of 2 limes
Salt and pepper to taste

In a large bowl, mix cucumber and watermelon. Add lime juice and toss well. Season with salt and pepper.

2 servings

DON'T DOUBT IT'S DELICIOUS SMOOTHIE

¼ cup peeled and cubed avocado
2 dates, pitted
¾ cup unsweetened almond milk
1½ scoops gluten-free protein powder
½ mango, peeled and cubed
1 cup filtered water
1 cup ice

Place all ingredients in a blender, and blend until rich and creamy.

1 serving

EASIEST BEEFIEST STIR-FRY

2 tablespoons olive oil, divided

Juice of 1 lemon

1 pound London broil, cut into strips

1 medium Vidalia onion, cut into chunks

1 yellow bell pepper, seeded and cut into chunks

½ head broccoli, cut into pieces

2 teaspoons gluten-free soy sauce, optional

Salt and pepper to taste

1 cup cooked brown rice

In a small bowl, combine 1 tablespoon olive oil and lemon juice. Add steak strips, cover bowl, and refrigerate for at least 30 minutes.

Remove from fridge, and allow steak to stand at room temperature for 30 minutes before cooking.

In a medium pan, heat ½ tablespoon olive oil over medium heat. Add onion, pepper, and broccoli, stirring frequently until barely softened. Remove from pan.

Add remaining olive oil to pan and turn heat to medium-high. Add beef strips, cooking for 2 to 3 minutes on each side. Add vegetable mixture and soy sauce if desired, and heat through. Add salt and pepper to taste.

Serve over brown rice.

2 servings

EASY FETA SCRAMBLE

1 teaspoon olive oil

1 cup chopped assorted low-carb vegetables

2 eggs, beaten

2 tablespoons goat or sheep feta cheese

Heat olive oil in small pan over medium heat. Add vegetables, stirring frequently until the vegetables have reached desired tenderness. Add eggs and stir constantly for 2 to 3 minutes. Add cheese and continue stirring until eggs are cooked and cheese has melted.

1 serving

EGGLESS EGG SALAD

1 pound extra-firm tofu

½ cup unsweetened Greek yogurt

1 red bell pepper, seeded and finely chopped

4 scallions, finely chopped

2 celery stalks, finely chopped

2 tablespoons chopped fresh parsley

1 tablespoon prepared Dijon mustard

3 teaspoons pickle relish

Salt and pepper to taste

2 cups mixed greens or 6 gluten-free crackers

In a large bowl, mash tofu. Add yogurt, pepper, scallions, celery, parsley, mustard, and relish. Mix very well and season with salt and pepper.

Serve on greens or with crackers.

2 lunch servings or 4 snack servings

EGGS IN A NEST

2 slices gluten-free bread
1 teaspoon olive oil
2 whole eggs
2 egg whites
Salt and pepper to taste
Hot sauce, optional

Cut a hole out of the center of each slice of bread using the rim of a small glass or a cookie cutter.

Heat olive oil in a small skillet over medium heat. Add bread and toast on one side.

In a small bowl, beat eggs and egg whites.

Turn bread over in skillet, and pour half of egg mixture into each hole. Cook until eggs are set, approximately 2 to 3 minutes. If desired, flip bread and cook for 2 to 3 more minutes.

Remove from pan, and season with salt and pepper. Top with hot sauce if desired.

2 servings

FAST 'N' EASY TURKEY AND BLACK BEAN SOUP

1 tablespoon olive oil

1 clove garlic, minced

1 small onion, chopped

½ tablespoon cumin

1 teaspoon dried oregano

½ teaspoon chili powder

½ pound ground turkey, browned, or 1½ cups cooked turkey, shredded

One 14-ounce can black beans, rinsed and drained

1 very large tomato, chopped

Salt and pepper to taste

In a medium saucepan, heat olive oil over medium heat. Add garlic and onion, stirring frequently until translucent. Add spices and stir well. Mix in turkey, beans, and tomato, and cook for an additional 10 to 12 minutes or until heated through. Season with salt and pepper.

2 servings

FAVORITE BROCCOLI

1 teaspoon salt

1 head broccoli, trimmed and cut into small chunks

2 tablespoons olive oil

½ large Vidalia onion, chopped

4 cloves garlic, chopped

1 to 2 tablespoons fresh oregano, chopped

Juice of ½ lemon

In a large pot, bring 2 cups water and salt to a boil. Add broccoli and lower heat, maintaining a low boil. Simmer until desired tenderness is reached.

Drain broccoli, reserving ¾ cup of liquid. Set broccoli aside.

In a large saucepan, heat olive oil over medium heat. Add onion and sauté until edges turn light brown. Add garlic and stir until softened, approximately 1 minute. Add broccoli and stir well. Stir in reserved liquid, oregano, and lemon juice. Mix well. Cook until veggies are heated through.

2 servings

GINGER POACHED CHICKEN

    4 cups organic chicken stock
    1-inch piece of fresh ginger root, peeled and cut into strips
    1 bay leaf
    1 small shallot, thinly sliced
    2 boneless skinless chicken breast halves
    6 scallions, chopped
    1 head endive, cut in quarters
    Salt and pepper to taste

Heat stock in a medium-sized saucepan over medium heat. Bring to a boil, and add sliced ginger. Reduce heat and simmer for five minutes. Add bay leaf and shallot slices. Simmer for 5 more minutes. Add chicken, scallions, and endive, and cook until chicken is tender, approximately 10 to 14 minutes. Season with salt and pepper.

2 servings

GREEN BEANS WITH ALMONDS

    ½ teaspoon salt
    1 pound green beans, ends trimmed
    1 teaspoon olive oil
    Salt and pepper to taste
    ⅓ cup slivered almonds

Fill a large pot ⅔ full with water and bring to a boil. Add salt and green beans. Cook until beans are bright green and desired tenderness is reached.

Drain beans and place in a bowl of cold water.

Drain beans a second time and place in a large bowl. Toss with olive oil and salt and pepper. Sprinkle with almonds and serve.

2 servings

GREEN BEANS WITH TOMATOES

1 tablespoon olive oil

1 medium onion, finely chopped

1 large tomato, chopped

1 pound green beans, ends trimmed

1 tablespoon chopped fresh basil

Salt and pepper to taste

In a large skillet, heat olive oil over medium heat. Add onion and stir until onion turns translucent. Add tomato and cook for 3 to 4 minutes until tomato softens. Add beans and bring mixture to a boil. Cover and reduce heat to low, stirring frequently until beans reached desired tenderness. Add basil and stir. Season with salt and pepper.

3 servings

GREEN VEGETABLE TRIO

2 cups broccoli florets

12 ounces okra, frozen or fresh

1 tablespoon olive oil

3 cloves garlic, minced

One 6-ounce jar chopped, marinated artichoke hearts

1½ tablespoons fresh lime juice

Steam broccoli florets; place in cold water and set aside.

Boil okra until limp. Drain and place in separate bowl to cool.

In a large sauté pan, heat olive oil over medium heat. Add garlic and cook for 2 to 3 minutes, taking care not to let garlic burn. Add artichoke hearts and cook for 3 to 5 minutes or until heated through. Add broccoli and okra and mix well. Stir occasionally until entire mixture is heated through. Remove from heat and sprinkle with lime juice.

2 servings

HERB-CRUSTED SALMON

1 tablespoon olive oil

1 pound salmon filet, cut into four pieces

2 tablespoons prepared Dijon mustard

Salt and pepper to taste

½ cup finely chopped fresh herbs of your choice (thyme, rosemary, oregano, basil, or parsley)

Preheat oven to 375 degrees.

Lightly brush a baking sheet with olive oil.

Spread meat side of filets with mustard and season with salt and pepper. Press herbs into each filet using your fingers or the back of a spoon. Place filets on baking sheet skin side down.

Bake for 7 to 10 minutes, or until desired doneness is reached.

3 servings

HOMEMADE TURKEY PATTIES

1 pound ground turkey
4 egg whites
¼ cup minced scallions
⅔ cup dried parsley
⅜ teaspoon dried marjoram
Salt and pepper to taste
½ tablespoon olive oil

Crumble turkey into a large mixing bowl. Mix in egg whites, scallions, parsley, and marjoram. Season with salt and pepper.

Shape turkey mixture into 12 small patties.

In a large skillet, heat olive oil and add patties. Cook for 5 to 6 minutes on each side or until cooked through.

Leftovers freeze well.

12 servings

KICKY CAULIFLOWER

½ head cauliflower, trimmed and broken into florets
Juice of 2 lemons
1 tablespoon olive oil
Pinch of red pepper flakes (more or less to taste)

Steam cauliflower until desired tenderness is reached.

Combine lemon juice, olive oil, and red pepper flakes in large bowl. Add cauliflower and toss to coat.

Serve warm or cold.

2 servings

KRUNCHY KALE

1 tablespoon olive oil

½ medium yellow onion, finely chopped

2 cloves garlic, minced

1 tablespoon prepared Dijon mustard

2 teaspoons apple cider vinegar

1 cup low-sodium, gluten-free organic chicken broth

4 cups kale, rinsed and torn into bite-sized pieces

2 tablespoons dried cranberries

Salt and pepper to taste

3 tablespoons sliced almonds

In a large pot, heat olive oil over medium heat. Add onion and garlic, stirring frequently until onion turns translucent, approximately 4 to 6 minutes. Stir in mustard, vinegar, and broth. Turn heat to high and bring mixture to a boil. Add kale pieces. Cover and cook until kale wilts, approximately 5 minutes. Add cranberries and continue boiling until cranberries have softened, approximately 15 minutes.

Remove from heat, and season with salt and pepper. Sprinkle with almonds before serving.

3 servings

LAMB BURGERS

For the Cucumber Yogurt Sauce:
   1 seedless cucumber, peeled
   2 tablespoons chopped fresh mint
   1½ teaspoons chopped garlic
   1½ tablespoons fresh lemon juice
   Salt and pepper to taste
   1 cup plain nondairy Greek yogurt

For the Burgers:
   1 pound ground lamb
   1 cup chopped white mushrooms
   ½ cup chopped onion
   1½ teaspoons finely chopped garlic
   ½ teaspoon ground cumin
   ⅓ cup crumbled feta
   Salt and pepper to taste

To make the sauce: Cut cucumber in half lengthwise and scoop out center seeds. Grate or finely chop, until you have approximately 1½ cups of grated cucumber.

Place cucumber in a mixing bowl with mint, garlic, lemon juice, salt and pepper, and yogurt. Mix together well and refrigerate.

To make the burgers: In a medium bowl, mix together lamb, mushrooms, onion, garlic, cumin, and feta. Form mixture into four patties, approximately 1 inch thick.

Spray a large skillet with cooking spray and heat over medium-high heat. Add patties and cook for 4 minutes. Reduce heat to medium and flip patties, cooking for an additional 1 to 2 minutes or until meat reaches desired doneness.

Place burgers on plates and top each with ¼ of the cucumber yogurt sauce.

4 servings

LEMON SHRIMP

Juice of 6 lemons

1 tablespoon gluten-free soy sauce

1 tablespoon cornstarch

1 pound shrimp, cleaned

1 tablespoon sesame oil

4 scallions, chopped

In a small bowl, mix lemon juice and soy sauce together. Add cornstarch and mix until a paste is formed. Add shrimp and toss to coat.

Heat sesame oil in a large skillet over medium-high heat. Add shrimp and cook for 6 to 8 minutes, until shrimp are cooked through.

Transfer to four serving plates, and garnish with scallions.

4 servings

MELON SMOOTHIE

½ cup unsweetened almond milk

⅓ cup peeled and cubed cantaloupe

2 tablespoons flaxseed

1 scoop gluten-free protein powder

¼ teaspoon gluten-free vanilla extract

½ cup ice

Place all ingredients in a blender, and blend until rich and creamy.

1 serving

MEXICAN TURKEY BURGERS

1 pound ground turkey breast

1 cup canned refried beans

3 garlic cloves, minced

3 tablespoons tomato paste

2 tablespoons chopped fresh cilantro

Salt and pepper to taste

1 jalapeño pepper, seeded and minced, optional

2 gluten-free rolls

Mix all ingredients except the rolls together. Shape into 4 patties. Cover and chill for 1 hour before cooking.

Grill or broil burgers for 3 to 4 minutes per side.

Serve open faced on ½ gluten-free roll.

4 servings

ORANGE CHICKEN SALAD

Juice of 2 lemons, divided

Juice of ½ orange

½ pound boneless, skinless chicken breasts, cut into bite-sized chunks

¼ cup plus 1 tablespoon olive oil

Salt and pepper to taste

4 cups mixed greens

2 stalks celery, chopped

½ orange, peeled and chopped

½ cup sliced almonds

In a small bowl, mix half of the lemon juice and the orange juice. Add chicken chunks and toss to coat. Cover and refrigerate for 1 hour.

In another small bowl, combine the remaining lemon juice, ¼ cup olive oil, and salt and pepper to create dressing.

In a large bowl, combine mixed greens, celery, orange, and almonds. Mix well.

Heat remaining olive oil in a medium sauté pan. Add chicken and sauté until cooked through.

Place cooked chicken on greens mixture and top with dressing.

2 servings

ORIENTAL TOFU STIR-FRY

8 ounces firm tofu

2 tablespoons safflower oil, divided

3 cloves garlic, minced

4 scallions, chopped

2 green chilies, deseeded and finely chopped

½ head Chinese cabbage, shredded

1 pound green beans, ends trimmed

4 ounces bean sprouts

4 tablespoons cashew butter

2 tablespoons gluten-free soy sauce

1½ cups unsweetened coconut milk

1 cup cooked brown rice

Cut tofu into 6 slices, and place each slice between paper towels to remove moisture. Slice into thin strips.

Heat 1 tablespoon safflower oil in a large pan over medium-high heat. Add tofu, stirring constantly for approximately 4 minutes, or until tofu is lightly browned. Remove tofu from pan.

Heat another tablespoon safflower oil in pan over medium-high heat. Add garlic, scallions, chilies, and cabbage and stir constantly for one minute. Add green beans and bean sprouts, continuing to stir for an additional 3 minutes. Lower heat to medium. Add cashew butter and soy sauce. Stir well, ensuring vegetables are coated. Add tofu and gently stir. Mix in coconut milk, and bring to a simmer. Simmer for 3 to 5 minutes, or until heated through.

Serve immediately over rice.

2 servings

PAN-GRILLED PORTOBELLO MUSHROOMS

4 large portobello mushrooms, de-stemmed

½ cup balsamic vinegar

½ cup gluten-free soy sauce

½ cup water

1 clove garlic, minced

2 sprigs fresh rosemary

1 teaspoon dried thyme

1 teaspoon dried oregano

1 tablespoon olive oil

Wash mushrooms and pat dry.

In a large bowl, combine vinegar, soy sauce, water, garlic, rosemary, thyme, and oregano. Stir well. Add mushrooms and toss to coat, ensuring that each one is covered well. Set aside to marinate for 30 minutes.

In a large skillet, heat olive oil over medium heat. Reserve marinade and place mushrooms in pan, top side down. Cook 3 to 4 minutes per side until lightly browned.

Meanwhile, remove rosemary sprigs from marinade. Pour marinade into pan and cover. Cook 6 to 8 more minutes or until mushrooms reach desired tenderness.

2 servings

PECAN LENTILS

2 cups low-sodium, gluten-free organic chicken broth

2 cups water

1 cup dried lentils

4 tablespoons pecan pieces

Salt and pepper to taste

In a medium saucepan, bring broth and water to a boil on high heat. Add lentils, stirring gently, and cover. Reduce heat to medium and simmer for 20 minutes.

While lentils are simmering, place pecan pieces on a flat baking sheet in toaster oven or under broiler for 2 to 4 minutes to toast, watching to ensure pecans do not burn.

Remove lid from saucepan and continue to cook lentils until liquid is absorbed.

Toss with pecans before serving and season with salt and pepper.

4 servings

PORK MEDALLIONS WITH APPLE RELISH

1½ tablespoons olive oil

One 1-pound pork loin, sliced into ¼-inch slices

2 medium Macintosh apples, cored and chopped

4 shallots, thinly sliced

5 tablespoons apple cider vinegar

Salt and pepper to taste

In a large skillet, slowly heat olive oil over medium heat. Add pork and brown each side, approximately 3 minutes per side, or until juice runs clear when pierced.

In a medium bowl, make relish by mixing together apples, shallots, and vinegar. Season with salt and pepper.

Place pork on serving plate and top with relish mixture.

3 servings

PROTEIN PANCAKES

2 cups gluten-free pancake and baking mix

½ cup soy, rice, or almond milk (or less for thinner pancakes)

3 large egg whites

2 scoops gluten-free protein powder

1 teaspoon gluten-free vanilla extract

½ teaspoon cinnamon (or more to taste)

½ cup pecans, chopped

2 teaspoons sunflower oil, divided

½ cup fresh berries

In a large mixing bowl, combine pancake mix, milk, egg whites, protein powder, vanilla, cinnamon, pecans, and 1 teaspoon sunflower oil. Mix well.

Using remaining sunflower oil, lightly coat a griddle or a flat pan. Warm pan over medium-high heat for 2 to 3 minutes, or until a drop of water sizzles when placed on it.

Measure ¼-cup servings of batter onto pan and cook. Flip pancakes when bubbles appear on the surface.

Top with berries and serve.

2 servings

PROTEIN POWERED OATMEAL

4 cups water

1 cup steel-cut gluten-free oats

½ apple, diced

2 tablespoons dates, chopped

2 tablespoons dried cranberries

4 tablespoons pecans, chopped

2 scoops gluten-free protein powder

¼ cup soy, almond, or rice milk

Stevia to taste

In a small saucepan, bring water to a boil. Add oats and stir. Reduce heat to low and simmer for 30 minutes.

Remove from heat and mix in fruit and nuts. Let cool for 5 minutes. Add protein powder and stir well.

Transfer to bowl, and mix with milk and stevia.

2 servings

QUICK AND DELICIOUS CHICKEN

1 tablespoon olive oil

4 boneless, skinless chicken breast halves

Salt and pepper to taste

1 onion, thinly sliced

3 plum tomatoes, cut into chunks

½ cup pitted green olives

⅓ cup chopped fresh cilantro

Juice of 1 lime

In a large skillet, heat olive oil over medium-low heat. Add chicken, season with salt and pepper, and cook until lightly browned and juices run clear, approximately 12 to 14 minutes.

Remove chicken from skillet and turn heat to medium. Add onion, stirring frequently until lightly browned. Add tomatoes and olives and cook for 3 more minutes, or until tomatoes have softened.

Remove pan from heat. Add cilantro and lime juice, and stir well.

Place chicken on plates, and top with tomato mixture.

4 servings

QUICK AND EASY LAMB CHOPS

Four 1-inch-thick lean lamb loin chops
1 clove garlic, minced
1 tablespoon minced fresh rosemary
1 teaspoon ground pepper
¼ cup organic honey
2 tablespoons dried mustard
Cooking spray

Preheat broiler.

Rub chops with garlic. Sprinkle each side with rosemary and pepper.

In a small bowl, combine honey and mustard. Set aside.

Spray a broiler pan with cooking spray. Place chops on broiler pan.

Broil chops approximately 5 inches from heat for 7 minutes. Turn chops and spread with honey mixture. Broil for an additional 6 to 8 minutes, or until meat has reached desired tenderness.

2 servings

QUICK CRAB CASSEROLE

½ pound cooked crabmeat

1 medium red bell pepper, seeded and chopped

½ cup green olives, diced

⅓ cup fresh cilantro, finely chopped

2 cloves garlic, minced

1 teaspoon chopped fresh basil

1 teaspoon chopped fresh oregano

Salt and pepper to taste

Pinch of cayenne pepper, optional

1 egg

1 cup gluten-free bread crumbs

1 cup soy yogurt

Juice of ½ lemon

1½ teaspoons olive oil

Preheat oven to 400 degrees.

In a large bowl, mix crab, pepper, olives, cilantro, garlic, basil, oregano, salt and pepper, and cayenne if desired.

In a medium bowl, mix egg, bread crumbs, yogurt, and lemon juice.

Gently mix egg mixture into crab mixture.

Lightly coat a 1-quart casserole dish with olive oil. Place crab mixture in casserole dish. Bake for approximately 20 minutes, or until lightly browned.

2 servings

QUINOA-STUFFED PEPPERS

1 cup water

1 cup quinoa

½ cup pecans, finely chopped

½ Granny Smith apple, peeled and chopped

Juice of ½ lemon

1 clove garlic, minced

3 tablespoons chopped fresh parsley

1 large tomato, chopped

Salt and pepper to taste

2 red bell peppers, de-seeded and cut in halves

1 tablespoon olive oil

Place water and quinoa in a small saucepan over medium heat. Cook until quinoa is tender, approximately 30 minutes.

In a large bowl, mix pecans, apple, lemon juice, garlic, parsley, and tomato. Add quinoa and season with salt and pepper. Fill each pepper half with ¼ quinoa mixture.

Lightly oil an 8" x 8" baking pan with olive oil. Fill pan with ¼ inch water. Place peppers in pan. Bake for 20 to 25 minutes, or until peppers are tender.

2 servings

RASPBERRY AVOCADO SMOOTHIE

1 ripe avocado, peeled, pitted, and cut into cubes

1 cup filtered water

1 cup raspberries

Juice of 1 orange

1 scoop gluten-free protein powder

Place all ingredients in a blender, and blend until smooth.

1 serving

ROASTED TURKEY BREAST

3 teaspoons minced fresh thyme

2 teaspoons grated lemon rind

3 cloves garlic, minced

1 turkey breast half, skin on (approximately 2 pounds)

1 tablespoon olive oil

4 sprigs fresh thyme

Preheat oven to 400 degrees.

In a small bowl, combine minced thyme, lemon rind, and garlic.

Loosen skin from turkey breast by using a small knife or your hand. Rub garlic mixture on turkey meat under the skin. Press skin back against meat.

Lightly coat a small broiling pan with olive oil. Place turkey skin side up in pan and sprinkle with the sprigs of thyme. If using a meat thermometer, insert into meaty part of breast, ensuring it is not resting against the bone. Bake for approximately 1½ hours, or until thermometer reaches 180 degrees.

Remove turkey from oven and let stand for 10 minutes before serving.

6 servings

ROSEMARY POACHED CHICKEN

2 boneless skinless chicken breast halves

2 cups low-sodium, gluten-free organic chicken broth

4 sprigs fresh rosemary or 2 teaspoons dried

Place chicken in single layer in a small pot. Cover with broth and herbs. Bring to a boil over medium heat. Reduce heat to low and simmer, covered, for 15 minutes.

Remove pan from heat and allow to sit for 15 minutes or until chicken is cooked through.

2 servings

SAFFRON CHICKEN

1 tablespoon olive oil

1 clove garlic, thickly sliced

2 boneless skinless chicken breast halves

2 shallots, thinly sliced

½ cup dry white wine

½ teaspoon saffron

2 tablespoons capers, drained

In a large pan, heat olive oil over medium heat. Add garlic and sauté until soft. Add chicken and sauté for 2 to 3 minutes on each side. Chicken should not brown.

Remove chicken from pan and set aside. Discard garlic.

Add shallots to pan and sauté until soft. Add wine and saffron, and cook for 2 minutes. Return chicken to pan, and cook until done, approximately 7 to 9 minutes.

Move chicken and sauce to serving bowl. Sprinkle with capers.

2 servings

SALMON ROLL-UP

2 tablespoons goat cheese spread
1 gluten-free tortilla
2 slices red onion
3 ounces smoked or fresh salmon
2 slices avocado

Spread goat cheese on tortilla. Arrange remaining ingredients on top.

Starting at one end, roll tortilla two times tightly, then fold long ends in toward center. Continue rolling tightly until complete.

1 serving

SAUTÉED ESCAROLE

1 tablespoon olive oil
2 garlic cloves, minced
2 heads escarole, trimmed, and leaves torn
Salt to taste
Juice of 1 lemon, optional

Heat olive oil in a large skillet over medium heat. Add garlic and stir constantly until lightly browned. Add escarole and season with salt. Cook, stirring frequently, until tender, approximately 12 minutes.

Serve immediately. Drizzle with lemon juice if desired.

3 servings

SLOW-ROASTED TOMATOES

4 plum tomatoes
Salt and pepper to taste
4 small sprigs thyme
1 clove garlic, sliced into 4 pieces
1 tablespoon olive oil, divided
½ tablespoon red wine vinegar

Preheat oven to 300 degrees.

Core each tomato and slice off bottom so tomato sits evenly. Season core hollow with salt and pepper. Insert 1 sprig thyme and 1 slice garlic into each hollow. Drizzle each tomato with several drops of olive oil.

Using remaining olive oil, lightly brush the inside of a small baking dish. Place tomatoes in baking dish. Bake tomatoes for approximately 90 minutes or until soft. Remove from oven.

Drizzle with vinegar just before serving.

2 servings

SPAGHETTI SQUASH DINNER

1 spaghetti squash, cut in half and seeded

1 tablespoon olive oil

1 small yellow onion, minced

4 cloves garlic, minced

1 pound ground turkey breast

2½ cups canned crushed tomatoes

3 tablespoons red wine

3 teaspoons capers, drained

3 teaspoons finely chopped fresh oregano

2 teaspoons crushed red pepper flakes

½ cup grated sharp soy, goat, or sheep cheese, optional

Preheat oven to 350 degrees.

Place squash skin side up on baking sheet and bake uncovered for 50 to 60 minutes, or until easily pierced with fork. When done, cool completely.

Using a large spoon, scoop out squash strands into a large bowl. (See note.)

Heat oil in a large skillet over medium-high heat. Add onion and garlic and sauté for 2 minutes. Add turkey, breaking it apart and stirring constantly for 3 more minutes. Add tomatoes and wine. Bring mixture to a boil, reduce heat to low, and simmer for 20 minutes. Add capers, oregano, and red pepper flakes, and simmer for an additional 5 minutes.

Pour turkey mixture on top of spaghetti squash, top with cheese if desired, and serve.

NOTE: Roasting squash can be done the day before. Refrigerate squash until ready to use. Heat thoroughly before completing last step of recipe.

2 servings

SPICY VEGGIE SMOOTHIE

6 large tomatoes

2 red or orange bell peppers

1 large zucchini

2 cloves garlic, minced

8 celery stalks

2 teaspoons ground flaxseed

Cayenne pepper to taste

1 tablespoon chili powder

1 scoop gluten-free protein powder

Juice of 1 lime, optional

Place tomatoes in a blender and process until smooth. Add remaining ingredients and blend until rich and creamy.

1 serving

STEAK WITH PARSLEY SAUCE

For the Sauce:
    1 clove garlic, cut into chunks
    1 cup loosely packed fresh parsley leaves
    ¼ cup olive oil
    Salt and pepper to taste

For the Steak:
    1 pound sirloin or strip steak
    1 tablespoon plus 1 teaspoon olive oil
    Salt and pepper to taste

To make the sauce: Puree all the ingredients in a blender until smooth. Set aside.

To make the steak: Brush both sides of the steak lightly with 1 teaspoon olive oil. Season with salt and pepper.

In large skillet, heat remaining olive oil over medium-high heat. Add steak and cook 4 to 5 minutes on each side, until browned lightly and desired doneness is reached.

Remove steak from pan and let stand for 10 minutes before slicing and topping with parsley sauce.

3 servings

STEAMED WHITE FISH

1 pound white fish (cod, haddock, or tilapia) cut into filets

Salt and pepper to taste

4 tablespoons rice vinegar

3 tablespoons gluten-free soy sauce

2 inches fresh ginger root, peeled and finely grated

6 scallions, green ends only, sliced into long thin pieces

Season both sides of fish filets with salt and pepper.

In a very large skillet over medium-high heat, combine vinegar, soy sauce, and ginger. Add fish to skillet and bring contents of pan to a boil. Cover and reduce heat to low. Simmer for 7 to 9 minutes or until fish is almost opaque. Add scallion slices and cover pan. Cook 2 to 3 more minutes until fish is cooked through.

3 servings

STEWED CHICKEN

2 tablespoons olive oil

4 bone-in chicken breasts halves

½ clove garlic, cut in half

1 red bell pepper, seeded and chopped

Zest of ½ orange

1 cup low-sodium, gluten-free organic chicken broth

½ cup fennel, thinly sliced

1 tablespoon dried basil

Salt and pepper to taste

16 Greek olives, pitted

In a Dutch oven, heat olive oil over medium heat. Add chicken and garlic and sauté, turning frequently until chicken browns, approximately 4 to 5 minutes per side. Remove garlic from pan and discard. Add pepper pieces and orange zest. Stir. Add broth, fennel, and basil. Season with salt and pepper. Cover, lower heat, and simmer until chicken is cooked through, approximately 30 to 35 minutes. Remove cover and stir in olives. Heat for 1 more minute.

4 servings

STIR-FRIED CHICKPEAS

2 tablespoons sunflower seeds

One 14-ounce can chickpeas, drained and rinsed

2 teaspoons chili powder

1 tablespoon safflower oil

2 cloves garlic, crushed

One 14.5-ounce can diced tomatoes

8 ounces fresh spinach, washed and tough stems removed

Salt and pepper to taste

Toast sunflower seeds by placing on a baking pan in oven or toaster oven at 400 degrees for approximately 5 minutes.

Place chickpeas in a medium bowl and toss with chili powder.

Heat safflower oil in a large sauté pan over medium heat. Add garlic and sauté until lightly browned. Add chickpeas and stir constantly for 2 minutes. Add tomatoes, with liquid, and spinach. Stir well and cook for 3 to 5 minutes or until spinach wilts and mixture is heated through. Season with salt and pepper.

2 servings

STRAWBERRY COCOA SMOOTHIE

½ cup silken tofu

½ cup unsweetened coconut milk

1 cup frozen strawberries

2 tablespoons unsweetened cocoa powder

1 tablespoon honey

Place all ingredients in a food processor and blend until smooth and creamy.

1 serving

STUFFED ZUCCHINI

4 large zucchini

1 teaspoon olive oil

1 medium onion, chopped

3 cloves garlic, minced

One 14-ounce can red kidney beans, rinsed and drained

1 tablespoon tomato paste

2 teaspoons chili powder

1 pound ground turkey breast

4 plum tomatoes, cut into 1-inch slices

Preheat oven to 375 degrees.

Cut zucchini in half lengthwise. Scoop out seeds and discard.

Place scooped-out zucchini shells in a large baking dish. Cover with boiling water. Let stand for 10 minutes. Drain zucchini and set aside.

In a medium sauté pan, combine oil, onion, garlic, beans, tomato paste, chili powder, and turkey. Stir and cook until turkey is cooked through and vegetables are soft.

Stuff the hollowed-out zucchini shells with turkey mixture. Cover with foil and bake for 30 minutes.

Remove from oven. Remove foil.

Place four to five slices of tomato onto each zucchini, and return to oven for an additional 8 to 12 minutes, or until zucchini is tender and filling is hot.

4 servings

SUPER SPEEDY SHRIMP SAUTÉ

1 tablespoon olive oil

5 cloves garlic, minced

1 pound shrimp

2 teaspoons chopped fresh basil

2 teaspoons chopped fresh oregano

Salt and pepper to taste

2 tablespoons white wine

1½ cups cooked brown rice

In a large sauté pan, heat olive oil over medium-high heat. Add garlic and sauté until softened. Add shrimp, stirring frequently for 2 minutes. Add basil, oregano, and salt and pepper. Stir well and add wine. Simmer for 2 to 3 minutes or until shrimp turns opaque.

Serve over rice.

3 servings

SUPER SPINACH SMOOTHIE

2 cups organic baby spinach

¼ cup arugula

2½ cups filtered water

¾ cup blueberries

1 peach, peeled and cut into chunks

1-inch piece fresh ginger root, peeled and diced

1 tablespoon ground flaxseed

1 tablespoon lemon rind

1 scoop gluten-free protein powder

1 cup ice

In a food processor, process spinach, arugula, and filtered water until well combined. Add remaining ingredients and process until smooth.

1 serving

TOMATO SALAD

3 tablespoons apple cider vinegar

2 tablespoons olive oil

¼ Vidalia onion, cut into very thin strips

3 teaspoons capers, rinsed and chopped

4 large tomatoes, chopped

Salt and pepper to taste

In a small bowl, whisk vinegar and olive oil together. Add onion and capers. Pour over tomatoes and season with salt and pepper.

4 servings

TOSSED GREENS WITH STRAWBERRIES

Juice of 1 large orange

2 tablespoons balsamic vinegar

1 teaspoon olive oil

4 cups mixed greens

2 tablespoons chopped scallions

1 cup sliced strawberries

In a medium bowl, combine orange juice, balsamic vinegar, and olive oil.

In a large bowl, gently toss together mixed greens, scallions, and strawberries.

Pour juice mixture over greens.

2 servings

TURKEY AND VEGETABLE PICCATA

1 pound turkey cutlets

2 teaspoons olive oil, divided

3 cups broccoli florets

3 cups sliced yellow summer squash

3 cloves garlic, minced

Salt and pepper to taste

1 cup low-sodium, gluten-free organic chicken broth

⅓ cup dry vermouth

1½ teaspoons grated lemon rind

Juice of ½ lemon

1 tablespoon capers, drained

Cut each turkey cutlet into four slices.

Warm 1 teaspoon olive oil in large skillet over medium heat. Add broccoli, summer squash, and garlic. Season with salt and pepper. Sauté vegetables until just tender. Remove vegetables from skillet and set aside.

Add remaining olive oil to skillet, turning heat to medium-high. Add turkey and cook for 2 to 3 minutes per side or until cooked through. Remove turkey from skillet and place on vegetable mixture.

Add broth, vermouth, and lemon rind to pan and bring to a boil. Scrape bottom of pan to release any browned vegetables or meat. Remove from heat and add lemon juice and capers.

Pour broth mixture over turkey and vegetables.

4 servings

TURKEY MANGO SALAD

Juice of 2 limes
1 tablespoon organic honey
2 tablespoons olive oil
1 teaspoon grated fresh ginger root
4 cups spinach leaves, tough stems removed
½ cup sliced jicama
½ cup diced radish
1 medium mango, peeled and cubed into bite-sized pieces
8 ounces cooked turkey, cubed

Place lime juice, honey, olive oil, and ginger root in a small covered container. Shake well.

In a large bowl, toss spinach, jicama, radish, mango, and turkey.

Pour dressing over turkey mixture and toss to coat.

2 servings

WARM CHICKEN SALAD

1 tablespoon chopped fresh tarragon

2-inch piece of fresh ginger root, peeled and finely chopped

4 tablespoons gluten-free soy sauce

2 boneless skinless chicken breast halves, cut into thin strips

1 tablespoon safflower oil

1 head Napa cabbage, chopped

¾ cup raw cashews

2 carrots, peeled and cut into matchsticks

8 to 10 romaine lettuce leaves, chopped

In a small bowl, mix tarragon, ginger, and soy sauce to make a marinade. Add chicken and mix. Cover and refrigerate for 2 to 4 hours.

In a large sauté pan, heat safflower oil over medium heat. Remove chicken from the marinade and place in pan. Stir chicken frequently until cooked through.

Combine cabbage, cashews, carrots, and romaine in a large bowl. Place cooked chicken mixture on top.

2 servings

WARM SPINACH SALAD

12 ounces baby spinach, rinsed well

1 small red onion, sliced in thin rings

¾ cup pine nuts

¼ cup olive oil

1 clove garlic, minced

1 cup balsamic vinegar

2 teaspoons molasses

Combine spinach, onion, and pine nuts in a large bowl.

In a medium saucepan, simmer olive oil and garlic for 5 minutes over low heat. Add vinegar and molasses, and turn heat to medium. Using a whisk, beat constantly until mixture boils. Remove from heat and let cool.

Pour dressing over spinach mixture.

4 servings

WHITE BEANS AND KALE

½ teaspoon olive oil

1 small onion, chopped

4 cups chopped kale

⅓ cup water

1 cup canned cannellini beans, rinsed and drained

2 plum tomatoes, chopped

½ teaspoon dried oregano

Pinch of salt

Heat olive oil in a large skillet over medium heat. Add onion and sauté until translucent. Add kale and water to skillet. Cover and reduce heat to low. Simmer until kale is wilted, approximately 5 to 7 minutes. Add beans, tomatoes, oregano, and salt. Uncover and cook until ingredients are heated through.

4 servings

ZINFANDEL CHICKEN

1 tablespoon plus 2 teaspoons olive oil

¾ teaspoon dried rosemary

¾ teaspoon dried basil

½ teaspoon dried thyme

1 clove garlic, minced

Salt and pepper to taste

4 boneless skinless chicken breast halves

1 teaspoon butter

2 shallots, sliced thinly

½ cup white Zinfandel wine

Combine 2 teaspoons olive oil, rosemary, basil, thyme, garlic, and salt and pepper in a small bowl, and mix well. Add chicken and toss to coat. Cover and marinate for approximately 15 minutes.

In large skillet, warm remaining olive oil over medium heat. Add chicken and cook until browned, approximately 6 minutes on each side. Add butter and shallots, and cook until shallots are brown and soft, approximately 6 to 8 minutes. Add wine and increase heat to medium-high. Cook for approximately 4 to 7 minutes, until wine reduces and chicken is cooked through.

4 servings

CONCLUSION

Go Forth and Balance!

Now that you have your Four-Week Plan for Hormonal Health, you may be wondering: what's next? How do you integrate all of this new information about diet, lifestyle, psychology, and attitude into your daily life—and how do you keep doing it week after week, month after month, year after year?

My answer to you is twofold and might at first seem contradictory: take it one day at a time . . . and think as far forward into the future as you can imagine.

I suggest taking one day at a time because at first making all these changes—or even a single change—can seem daunting, perhaps even overwhelming. If so, that's okay. Just take it step by step. Don't think about cutting out sugar for the rest of your life—just avoid it *today*. Don't worry about how you're going to avoid gluten or get in your daily workout or eat organic next week when you go to visit your folks for a holiday weekend. Just concentrate on following the Plan *today*. Many things that seem impossible for the long haul actually seem quite doable today . . . and then tomorrow . . . and then the next day. And if at first you can only imagine making a few small changes, start with where you are and don't worry about where you're going.

At the same time, I want to acknowledge that we're all tempted by instant gratification. But it's the long haul of what you do in life that really has the biggest consequences. When you're trying to choose between a serving of fresh berries and a slice of chocolate cake, that chocolate cake can sure look good! Let's face it—chocolate cake is delicious! It looks good, it smells good, it definitely tastes good, and right after you eat it, you feel terrific. Why *wouldn't* you choose it over the berries, every single time?

But if every time you have a choice, you choose the cake, over time, the effects of those choices accumulate—and therein lies the problem. Life is made up of hundreds of little choices, day after day after day. Any one choice might not make that much of a difference by itself. But in the long run, those choices add up, and they can have unbelievably dramatic consequences. One set of consequences might include PMS, painful periods, and a difficult transition to perimenopause, not to mention inflammation, fatigue, low sex drive, acne, headaches, irritability, mood swings, loss of concentration, lack of focus, anxiety, and depression. Another set of consequences might include clarity and focus, a sense of joy and well-being, feeling sexy and sensual, and enjoying seemingly boundless energy and vitality. The choice truly is up to you.

We are looking for progress, not perfection. If you make healthy choices 85 to 90 percent of the time, you can achieve fabulous results—I promise. It's hard to imagine what a huge impact your diet, your lifestyle, your thoughts, and your hormones can have on your health and well-being. That's why I hope you'll commit to this four-week plan—so you don't have to imagine the dramatic results. You'll be able to see them for yourself.

Would you like to have more energy for your children, your partner, and yourself? Would you like to have the mental focus and clarity that enables you to work at peak efficiency, and the sense of joy and well-being that allows you to savor every moment of your life? Would you like to be bounding out of bed every morning without an alarm, and going to sleep every night relaxed and ready to sleep deeply? Would you like to achieve your ideal weight, enjoy your sex life, and feel like yourself every single day of the month? All of this is possible for you. It just depends on the choices that you make.

So I'd like to leave you with one last thought: if you take care of your body, it takes care of you. It is truly unbelievable how much of a game changer this approach can be. If you eat the foods that support your body, if you get the exercise and sleep your body craves, if you lighten your toxic burden and release excessive stress, your body will reward you beyond measure. I wish you all the best on this next stage of your journey.

APPENDIX A
Snack List

Within the meal plan, I have recommended that you eat three meals and two snacks per day. Following is a list of snacks for you to choose from. With this, you can choose anything that sounds good to you at the point when you are going to eat it. Each of these is specially balanced to have the nutrition to fill you up and keep you satisfied throughout the day.

- 1 hard-boiled egg and 10 almonds
- ½ apple with 1 tablespoon cashew or almond butter
- ½ cup soy, goat, or sheep Greek-style yogurt with 2 tablespoons blueberries, raspberries, or strawberries
- 1 ounce sliced turkey and 1 ounce soy, goat, or sheep cheese on ½ gluten-free tortilla
- 2 ounces flaked salmon (fresh or canned) mixed with 1 tablespoon yogurt, a dash of lemon juice, and salt and pepper, served on 6 gluten-free crackers
- 2 ounces hummus with 1 cup sliced vegetables
- 3 ounces smoked salmon layered with 1 ounce soy cream cheese and 3 to 4 tomato slices, seasoned with salt and pepper to taste
- 1 cup mixed greens and 2 ounces sliced turkey or chicken topped with 1 tablespoon gluten-free dressing
- 1 unsweetened rice cake with 2 slices avocado
- 1 unsweetened rice cake with 1 tablespoon almond or cashew butter

APPENDIX B
Additional Supplementation

In addition to the supplements I laid out in the four-week plan, there is much you can do if you are struggling with issues such as mood fluctuations, anxiety, or even fibroids and endometriosis. If you are facing any of the issues listed below, please feel free to add these supplements to the program outlined in Chapter 8.

MOOD ISSUES

Try the following supplements one at a time, or check with your practitioner. Don't take any of these supplements if you are on antidepressants or an MAO inhibitor without checking with your practitioner.

- 5-HTP: 50 to 150 mg at night *or* SAMe: 400 to 1600 mg during the day
- Theanine: 100 to 200 mg during the day

STRESS AND ANXIETY

Breakfast:

- Serenagen: one tablet

Lunch:

- Serenagen: one tablet

Dinner:

- GABA: 500 mg taken with a quarter of an apple and about five nuts
- L-tryptophan: 500 mg taken with a quarter of an apple and about five nuts

Bedtime:

- Serenagen: one tablet

LIBIDO

- ArginMax (as directed) *or* Libido (as directed) *or* maca: 1.5 to 3 grams per day

CRAVINGS

- Chromium picolinate: 100 to 200 mcg per day taken before meals
- 5-HTP: 50 to 100 mg per day taken at night
- Theanine: 100 to 200 mg per day

PREMENSTRUAL SYNDROME (PMS)

Breakfast:

- Evening Primrose oil: 500 mg
- L-carnitine: 500 mg per day
- Taurine: 1000 mg per day
- A proprietary blend of chromium picolinate, black cohosh, wild yam, lemon balm, burdock, chasteberry, dong quai, and maca

Lunch:

- Evening primrose oil: 500 mg
- Vitamin A/beta-carotene: 5000 to 8000 IU
- B-complex with 50 to 100 mg of B6: once daily
- Vitamin E, mixed tocoperhols: 400 to 800 mg per day

Dinner:

- Evening primrose oil: 500 mg
- Optional: Topical progesterone cream: ¼ teaspoon on inner wrist from day 14 of cycle to menses

PAINFUL PERIODS

Breakfast:

- Evening primrose oil: 500 mg

Lunch:

- Evening primrose oil: 500 mg

Dinner:

- Evening primrose oil: 500 mg

PERIMENOPAUSE

- A proprietary blend of red clover extract, ashwagandha extract, passionflower extract, chaste tree extract, kudzu extract, wild yam extract, black cohosh extract

ENDOMETRIOSIS

Avoid all dairy products and red meat, unless organic, and reduce intake of saturated fats. Avoid environmental and food toxins. Maintain a healthy body weight without excess body fat and get moderate exercise. Make sure to have a healthy gut to help with detoxification, which you can do by avoiding sugar, alcohol, preservatives, and hydrogenated and trans fats, as well as eating plenty of fiber and fresh vegetables.

If your digestive symptoms do not resolve, work with a functional medicine practitioner.

Breakfast:

- Alpha lipoic acid: 500 to 1000 mg
- Pycnogenol: 30 mg

Lunch:

- B complex with 100 mg of B6
- Vitamin A/beta-carotene: 5000 IU
- Omega-6: 500 to 1500 mg
- Vitamin C: 1000 mg
- Vitamin E: 400 IU

Dinner:

- Pycnogenol: 30 mg
- Selenium: 50 to 200 mcg

Bedtime:

- Progesterone cream: ¼ teaspoon on the inside of wrist from day 14 through menses

FIBROIDS

Avoid all dairy products and red meat, unless organic, and reduce intake of saturated fats. Avoid environmental and food toxins. Reduce intake of caffeine and unhealthy fats, such as trans fats and saturated fats. Add iodine to your diet in the form of seaweed. Maintain a healthy body weight without excess body fat and get moderate exercise. Make sure to have a healthy gut to help with detoxification, as suggested on page 236. If your digestive symptoms do not resolve, work with a functional medicine practitioner.

Breakfast:

- Evening primrose oil: 500 mg
- Alpha lipoic acid: 300 mg
- L-carnitine: 1000 to 1500 mg
- CoQ10: 100 mg or, if you're over 40, Ubiquinol: 100 mg
- GLA: 250 to 720 mg
- Inositol: 500 mg

Lunch:

- Evening primrose oil: 500 mg

Dinner:

- Evening primrose oil: 500 mg
- NAC: 600 mg *or* milk thistle 100 to 200 mg

Bedtime:

- Calcium: 500 to 1000 mg per day
- Magnesium, half the amount of calcium: 250 to 500 mg per day
- Progesterone cream, as directed on package

POLYCYSTIC OVARIAN SYNDROME (PCOS)

Maintain a healthy body weight without excess body fat. It's important to keep blood sugar stable by eating small, frequent meals and following the dietary recommendations of the 28-day plan. Many products are available to help with glucose regulation, including UltraMeal Plus 360. The recommended dose for that product is two scoops twice daily. It can also be used as breakfast if supplemented with 1000 to 2000 mg per day of fish oil EPA/DHA or the following supplements:

Breakfast:

- Alpha lipoic acid: 200 to 600 mg
- Biotin: 4 to 8 mg
- Chromium picolinate: 600 to 1200 mcg
- CLA: 1000 to 3000 mg
- Taurine: 1000 to 3000 mg

Lunch:

- Vitamin D: Have your levels tested and work with a practitioner to make sure they are optimal. Most people need to supplement with 1000 to 2000 IU per day.

- B-complex with 100 mg of B6

- Manganese: 5 to 10 mg

Bedtime:

- Magnesium: 400 to 800 mg per day

- Vitamin C: 1000 to 4000 mg per day

- Vitamin D: 1000 to 2000 mg per day—and make sure to check vitamin D levels

- Zinc: 25 to 50 mg per day

FOR ADRENAL SUPPORT, SEE *IS IT ME OR MY ADRENALS?*

APPENDIX C

Symptoms of Premenstrual Syndrome

Aches and pains, including backache

Adult acne

Alcohol sensitivity

Anxiety

Asthma

Bleeding gums

Bloating

Bone loss

Breast pain or tenderness

Bruising

Changes in appetite

Clumsiness

Confusion

Cramps

Cravings

Crying spells or tearfulness

Depression

Diarrhea or constipation

Dizziness

Drowsiness

Dry skin

Eye pain

Facial swelling

Fatigue

Fear of going out alone

Fear of losing control

Feeling depressed or overwhelmed

Fibroids

Forgetfulness or poor memory

Fuzzy thinking or difficulty concentrating

Hair loss

Headaches

Heart palpitations

Herpes or cold sores

Hives or rashes

Hot flashes and night sweats

Indecision

Inefficiency

Insomnia or restless sleep

Irregular periods

Leg cramps

Leg swelling

Low libido

Lowered productivity

Mood swings, irritability, rage

Nausea or vomiting

Panic attacks

Poor coordination

Poor judgment

Poor vision or visual changes

Restlessness or tension

Seizures

Sensitivity to light and noise

Social withdrawal

Sore throat

Spots in front of eyes

Stiffness or joint pain

Suspiciousness

Swollen fingers

Unwanted hair growth

Urinary dysfunction and/or bladder irritation

Vaginal dryness

Weight gain

APPENDIX D

Modifying Current
and Historical Stress

Following are a number of approaches that I recommend for addressing current and historical stress. Glance over the list and see which of them appeals most to you. You might even find two or three that you would like to try.

- *Massage.* For treating yourself to an hour or two of down time, there is nothing like a good massage! Many different types are available at spas and gyms, or you might look for ads at local health-food stores, yoga studios, or dance studios. Another option is to buy a good book on do-it-yourself massage and then do a massage exchange with a romantic partner or a friend.

- *Acupuncture and acupressure.* This ancient Chinese healing technique can be a wonderful way to relax and restore your energy and sense of well-being. Acupuncture relies on tiny, hair-thin needles, which don't hurt, while acupressure involves pressure at key points. Look online for an accredited practitioner.

- *Yoga.* There are many different yoga styles. Some focus on relaxation and restoration, while others are oriented more toward exercise and vigorous workouts. A good beginning restorative yoga class does not require you to be in shape or even to exert yourself—and you may begin to feel the benefits immediately.

- *Tai chi.* Tai chi is a Chinese "moving meditation" technique that involves moving very slowly from pose to pose. Like yoga, some forms are gentle and restorative, while others are more vigorous and recall the practice's history as a martial art. Depending on which class you take, you might consider it exercise, relaxation—or both!

- *Qigong.* Pronounced "chi gung," this is an ancient Chinese martial art that is also used for its healing properties. Like the others, it contributes to relaxation, health, and well-being, as well as providing for many people a personal spiritual connection.

- *Chiropractic.* This discipline involves realignment of the spine to restore the body's natural energy. It might help to liberate any emotional memories that are locked within your body, perhaps supplemented by talk therapy or other forms of emotional work. (For more information, see http://nccam.nih/gov/chiropractic.)

- *Feldenkrais.* The official name for this practice is the Feldenkrais Method of Somatic Education. The goal is to learn natural movement, conservation of energy, and freedom from rigid ideas about yourself. (For more information, see www.feldenkrais.com.)

- *Guided imagery.* Research shows that this approach can help you break free of long-held patterns of thought to find greater emotional freedom. Guided imagery draws on your memory and imagination of experiences involving sight, sound, smell, and touch. (For more information, see www.belleruthnaparstek.com and www.healthjourneys.com.)

- *Hypnosis or self-hypnosis.* Many people use this technique—either solo or with a licensed practitioner—to overcome unwanted habits or to alter unwanted emotions, such as phobias and the trauma that comes from painful memories. Hypnosis can also be extremely useful in treating chronic pain. (For more information, see www.natboard.com.)

- *Polarity therapy.* This technique focuses on rebalancing your energy by identifying places where your energy is blocked, unbalanced, or "frozen" into a fixed pattern. Many people find it useful in freeing themselves from painful or traumatic past experiences. (For more information, see www.polaritytherapy.org.)

- *The Relaxation Response.* Pioneered by Harvard internist Herbert Benson, this approach involves reaching a state of deep relaxation to overcome pain, anxiety, and stress. Many people find it useful for both physiological and psychological problems. (For more information, see www.relaxationresponse.org.)

- *Rolfing.* Founded by Ida P. Rolf, this technique opens up areas of the body that had previously been clenched in tension, releasing emotional memories and associations as well. (For more information, see www.rolf.org.)

- *Integrative Manual Therapy (IMT).* Physical and emotional relief is the goal of this technique, which uses gentle manipulative techniques to relieve pain. (For more information, see www.centerimt.com.)

- *Music therapy.* Music therapy relies on the healing, evocative power of music as you listen to music, write songs, perform music, and improvise sounds. This approach may be able to reach you in places where your rational, verbal self may be unwilling to go, helping you free yourself from emotional baggage. (For more information, see www.musictherapy.org.)

- *Art therapy.* By tapping into your creative, expressive side, art therapy helps you explore emotions in a nonverbal way so that you can release past trauma and move forward with greater freedom. (For more information, see www.arttherapy.org.)

- *Dance and movement therapy.* Dance and movement can be very helpful in freeing yourself from painful emotions locked in your body and your unconscious mind. (For more information, see www.adta.org.)

- *Pet therapy.* Owning a pet, horseback riding, or other contact with animals can be deeply healing and de-stressing. (For more information, see www.healthline.com/galecontent/pet-therapy.)

- *Emotional Freedom Techniques.* Founded by nondenominational minister Gary Craig, this approach involves tapping certain key points with your fingertips to release emotional and physical stress while rebalancing your energy. (For more information, see www.eftuniverse.com.)

- *Eye Movement Desensitization and Reprocessing: EMDR.* This comprehensive approach involves many different therapies, including psychodynamic, cognitive-behavioral, interpersonal, experiential, and body-centered techniques. The power of the approach comes from integrating body, mind, and emotions. (To learn more, see http://emdria.org.)

- *The Work of Byron Katie.* This powerful cognitive technique involves questioning some of your most painful and deeply held beliefs about yourself, such as "I'm not attractive," "I'll never find someone to love me," or "My life will never get better." The Work invites you to ask yourself whether these debilitating beliefs are really true and then helps you release them. (For more information, see www.thework.com.)

- *Twelve-Step support groups.* These groups can be extremely useful for anyone who has been closely involved with an alcoholic or a person with an addiction, either in childhood or adulthood. Two of the best-known such groups are Al-Anon, for the loved ones of alcoholics, and ACOA (Adult Children of Alcoholics), for those who grew up with alcoholic or addicted parents and caretakers. (For more information, go to www.12step.org.)

- *The Hoffman Institute Quadrinity Process.* This is an eight-day intensive course that incorporates automatic writing, guided visualizations, and many other experiential techniques to help you release painful experiences from the past. I personally have engaged in this process, and I currently serve on its board because I believe so strongly in how helpful it can be. (For more information, see www.hoffmaninstitute.org.)

RESOURCES

CLINICAL LABORATORIES

I rely on the following clinical laboratories for much of my diagnostic testing. You should work with an integrative or functional medical practitioner in getting tested.

- Aeron LifeCycles Clinical Laboratory (www.aeron.com): Adrenal testing/ hormone panel, one of the few labs accepted in the state of New York

- Alletess Medical Laboratory (www.foodallergy.com): Tests for food allergies, food sensitivities, and seasonal allergies

- Diagnos-Techs (www.diagnostechs.com): Adrenal testing, hormonal/ digestive testing

- Doctor's Data (www.doctorsdata.com): Tests for heavy metal toxicity, digestive issues, and adrenal function

- Genova Diagnostics (http://www.gdx.net): Tests genetic profile, adrenal function, comprehensive parasitology, allergies, amino acid deficiency, stool testing, and liver detoxification

- Metametrix Clinical Laboratory (www.metametrix.com): Tests for amino acid deficiency, allergies, stool, digestive issues, and toxic burden

- NeuroScience (www.neurorelief.com): Tests neurotransmitter levels, amino acids, adrenal function, hormones, and vitamin D level

- ZRT Laboratory (www.zrtlab.com): Tests hormonal function, vitamin D level, and cardiometabolic markers

COMPOUNDING PHARMACIES

- Professional Compounding Centers of America PCCA (www.pccarx.com)

How to Find Compounding Pharmacists

- International Academy of Compounding Pharmacists (http://www.iacprx.org)

- Emerita Progesterone Cream (www.emerita.com)

COSMETICS, BATH, AND BEAUTY

Listed below are products that don't contain parabens, dyes, lead, or other toxins. It's best to choose fragrance-free products. For more information on personal care products, check out these websites:

- The Environmental Working Group (www.ewg.org)

- The Campaign for Safe Cosmetics (www.safecosmetics.org)

Air and Water Filters

- Bathtub and showerhead filters (www.santeforhealth.com)

- Custom Pure water purification systems (www.custompure.com)

- New Wave Enviro bathtub and shower filters (www.enviroproductsinc.com)

- Kenmore Reverse Osmosis Drinking Water System (www.sears.com/kenmore-reverse-osmosis-drinking-water-system/p-04238156000P)

- PiMag Ultra Shower System (www.nikken.com)

Chemical-Free Mini/Maxi Pads, Reusable Cups, and Tampons

These companies offer usable and chemical-free hygiene products:

- GladRags (www.gladrags.com)

- Goddess Moons (www.goddessmoons.com)

- Natracare (www.natracare.com)

Gluten-Free Cosmetics

- Gluten-Free Hub (www.glutenfreehub.com)
- Mirage Lip Gloss (www.miragelipgloss.com)

Hair Products

- By the Planet (www.bytheplanet.com)
- EcoColors (www.ecocolors.net)
- Infinite Health Resources (www.infinitehealthresources.com): safe hair dyes
- Intelligent Nutrients (www.intelligentnutrients.com): safe hair dyes
- La Bella Gelle, La Bella Hair Mist, and La Bella Mousse (www.labellamaria.com)
- Lotus Brands (www.lotusbrands.com)
- Louise Galvin (www.louisegalvin.com)
- Max Green Alchemy (www.maxgreenalchemy.com)
- Morrocco Method International (www.morroccomethod.com)
- Suki skin care (www.sukiskincare.com)
- Sunrise Lane (www.sunriselaneproducts.com): safe hair dyes

Sunscreens

- Natural Mineral Sunscreen SPF 30 (www.saffronrouge.com)
- Aubrey Organics (www.aubrey-organics.com)
- Badger SPF 15 for Face and Body (www.badgerbalm.com)
- Burt's Bees Chemical-Free Sunscreen SPF 15 and SPF 30 (www.burtsbees.com)
- Kiss My Face Sunscreens (www.kissmyface.com)
- Soléo Organics Sunscreen (www.soleoorganics.com)

EXERCISE AND HEALING PRODUCTS

Workout and Exercise Products

- Biofeedback: EmWave Personal Stress Reliever (www.heartmathstore.com/category/emwaveworks)
- Fredrick Hahn's Serious Strength Slowburn Personal Training Studios (www.seriousstrength.com)
- JJ Virgin's 4x4 Workout (www.jjvirgin.com/4x4workout-dvds)
- The Slow Burn Home Workout DVD (www.slowburnfitness.com)
- X-iser (www.xiser.com): great exercise for short interventions

Light Therapy Products

- BioBrite (www.biobrite.com)
- The SunBox Company (www.sunbox.com)

FOOD

Gluten-free Products

You can obtain gluten-free foods from the following sources:

Abigail's Bakery
352 Sugar Hill Road
Weare, NH 03281
(603) 724-6544
www.abigailsbakery.com

Against the Grain Gourmet
22 Browne Court, Unit 119
Brattleboro, VT 05301
(802) 258-3838
www.againstthegraingourmet.com

Sami's Bakery
2399 E. Busch Blvd.
Tampa, FL 33612
(877) 989-2722
www.samisbakery.com/

Mediterranean snacks, lentil crackers, and chips: (www.mediterraneansnackfoods.com)

Elaine's Pantry (www.elainespantry.com)

For more information on gluten and gluten-free products, check out the following Websites:

- www.wisegeek.com/what-is-gluten.htm
- www.glutenfreeworks.com/gluten-disorders/gluten
- www.gicare.com/diets/gluten-free-diet

A number of gluten-free foods are available. Here I list some brands and products that I have personally used. You can find these and other brands at a natural foods store or by ordering online at www.glutenfree.com or www.glutenfreemall.com. Be mindful, though, that a product being gluten free does not ensure that all of its ingredients are healthy and safe for you, so check the labels carefully.

Bagels and Breads

- Against the Grain Gourmet sesame bagels
- Better Bread pizza
- Blue Diamond Nut Thins crackers
- Enjoy Life bagels
- Food for Life raisin pecan bread
- Glutino frozen bagels, breadsticks (pizza and sesame), biscuits, and original crackers
- Mary's Gone Crackers (all flavors)

Cereal

- Bakery on Main apple raisin cereal
- Cream Hill Estates Lara's Rolled Oats
- Nature's Gate Mesa Sunrise

Condiments

- Barkat vegetable gravy mix
- Esparaggo's asparagus guacamole
- Hempzels horseradish hemp and honey mustard
- J & S Peabutter (nonpeanut butter)
- Maxwell's Kitchen chicken gravy
- Mr. Spice Indian curry sauce

Desserts

- Arico Chocolate Chip Cookie Bar
- Barkat waffle ice cream cones
- Candy Tree black licorice vines
- EnviroKidz cookies
- Eragrain frozen natural oatmeal raisin cookies
- Glutino Shortcake Dreams

Entrees

- Amy's frozen entrees
- Chebe frozen pizza
- George's pizza
- Gillian's frozen pizza
- Glutino frozen pizza
- Mrs. Leeper's hamburger entrees

Grains

- Shiloh Farms brown basmati rice
- Shiloh Farms kasha
- Shiloh Farms millet

Mixes

- Authentic Foods chocolate cake mix
- Authentic Foods pancake and baking mix
- Betty Crocker gluten-free brownies
- 'Cause You're Special cake mix
- 'Cause You're Special sugar cookie mix
- Namaste baking mixes
- Pamela's Pantry baking and pancake mix
- The Cravings Place all-purpose pancake and waffle mix

Pasta

- Ancient Harvest quinoa linguine
- Ancient Harvest quinoa pasta elbows
- Glutino macaroni
- Tinkyada brown rice pasta (all shapes)—my favorite!
- Tinkyada organic brown rice pasta (all shapes)
- Tinkyada spinach brown rice spaghetti
- Tinkyada vegetable brown rice spirals

Snacks

- Barkat sesame pretzels
- EnviroKidz rice bars
- Glutino pretzels

Soups

- Celefibr vegetarian bouillon cubes
- Full Flavor Foods chicken soup stock

Yeast-Free Flour

- Bob's Red Mill gluten-free flour

GMO-Free Food

I personally recommend avoiding genetically modified foods if possible, so I'm providing you the following list of companies that offer GMO-free products: **Baking Mixes, Flours, Bread, Baked Goods**

- Arrowhead Mills
- Bob's Red Mill
- French Meadow Bakery
- Grindstone Bakery
- Pamela's Products
- To Your Health Sprouted Flour Co.

Dairy—organic when possible

- Brown Cow plain yogurt
- FAGE yogurt
- The Greek Gods yogurt
- Pure Indian Foods ghee
- Stonyfield Farm yogurt—no sugar

Meats, Vegetables

- US Wellness meats
- Wisconsin Healthy Grown potatoes

Prepared Foods (Soups, Canned Goods, Soy Sauce, Frozen Entrées)

- Amy's Kitchen
- Annie's Naturals
- Cascadian Farm
- Eden Foods
- Genisoy
- Imagine Foods
- Lundberg Family Farms
- Muir Glen
- Natural Choice Foods
- Purity Foods
- San-J
- Spectrum Organic Products
- Thai Kitchen
- Tradition Miso
- Vitasoy
- WhiteWave
- Whole Foods Market products

Snacks, Salsas, Chips, Desserts

- Barbara's Bakery
- Bearitos
- Clif Bar
- Garden of Eatin'
- Kettle Brand chips
- Nature's Path
- Purity Foods
- Que Pasa
- Zukay Live Foods

Medical Foods

- UltraMeal Plus 360, available through Metagenics

Organic Food Sources

- Organic Chocolate (www.dagobachocolate.com)

- EatWild (eatwild.com)

- Alaskan Seafood (alaskaseafoodcompany.com)

- For chia seeds: www.nuts.com/cookingbaking/chia-seeds

- For green drinks: www.healthygreendrink.com

- US Wellness Meats (www.uswellnessmeats.com)

HOUSEHOLD PRODUCTS

Following is a list of my favorite nontoxic kitchen, bed, and bath products. I have tried to find you products that are attractive, durable, and easy to find at your local natural foods store or on the Internet. I use these products at my clinic and in my home and to the best of my knowledge they are as green as they claim to be. You can also search for products in the Gaiam catalog (www.gaiam.com) and the Whole Earth Catalog (www.wholeearth.com), both of which are great resources for nontoxic— or at least, less toxic—home products. Another great resource is Seventh Generation (www.seventhgeneration.com).

Cleaning Products

Fruit and Vegetable Washes

- Environné fruit and vegetable wash (www.environne.com)

- FIT fruit and vegetable wash, Organiclean, and Vegi-Clean (www.fitwash.com)

- Women to Women website for nontoxic cleaning recipes (www.womentowomen.com/detoxification/nontoxic-greencleaning-page2.aspx)

Heat and Therapy Packs

- Grandpa's Garden herbal heat packs (www.grandpasgarden.com)

Household Cleaning Products

- Citrus Magic (www.beaumontproducts.com)

- Environmentally safe, energy efficient products: www.greenstore.com

- Earth Friendly Products (http://ecos.com)

- Mrs. Meyer's Clean Day (www.mrsmeyers.com)

Mold

- To remove mold that won't disappear with a good dosing of tea tree oil: www.toxicmoldadvisor.com

- Seventh Generation dishwashing liquids (www.seventhgeneration.com)

Household and Bedroom Products

Air Filters

- Air Wellness Power Pro and Traveler (www.nikken.com)

- Austin Air Healthmate (www.austinairstore.com)

- Nordic Pure air filters (www.airfiltershome.com)

Hypoallergenic Bedding

- Allergy-free and asthma bedding: www.allergyasthmatech.com

- Allergy-proof mattress and pillow covers: www.allergystore.com

Whole-System Water Filters

- Kinetico 1030 and 1060 de-chlorinators (www.kinetico.com)

Kitchenware

Blenders

- Vitamix blender (www.vitamix.com)

Glass Storage Containers

- Crate and Barrel rectangular storage containers (www.crateandbarrel.com)

- Pyrex round and rectangular storage containers (www.pyrex.com)

Nonleaching Baking Pans

- Cabela's cast-iron skillets (www.cabelas.com)

- Pyrex glass baking pans (www.pyrex.com)

Rice Cookers/Pressure Cookers with Stainless Steel Parts

- Miracle stainless steel rice cooker (www.ultimate-weight-products.com)

- Small ceramic rice cooker/crock pressure cooker (www.kushistore.com)

Stainless Steel Water Bottles

- Enviro Products (www.enviroproductsinc.com)

Tap/Drinking Water Filters

- K5 drinking water station (www.kinetico.com)

- PiMag: Aqua Pour, Aqua Pour Deluxe, Aqua Pour Express, deluxe under-counter water system, countertop water system, Optimizer (www.nikken.com)

- Water filters: www.custompure.com

MEDICAL THERAPIES

Biodentistry

Many chronic health problems may have been caused by damage from the mercury in dental fillings, root canals, and untreated tooth decay. Biological dentists are trained to recognize the close connection between dental health and body structure, the immune and nervous systems, and nutrition.

Try these resources to find a practitioner near you:

- Huggins Applied Healing (www.hugginsappliedhealing.com/find-dentist.php)

- www.mercuryfreedentists.com

- Foundation for Toxic Free Dentistry (www.toxicfreedentistry.com)

Functional Medicine

Functional medicine is a comprehensive approach to health care that treats the whole patient first, not the disease. It integrates the best of Western and ancient modalities, with an emphasis on maintaining organ integrity and subtly shifting core physiology through nutrition and lifestyle.

Contact this organization to find a functional medical practitioner near you:

- The Institute for Functional Medicine (www.functionalmedicine.org)

Homeopathy

- National Center for Homeopathy (www.nationalcenterforhomeopathy.org)

Hormone Replacement Therapy—Bioidentical Hormones

Hormone therapy replenishes the hormones your body needs to function properly using bioidentical hormones. BodyLogicMD's affiliated physicians are highly trained in natural bioidentical hormone therapy integrated with nutrition and fitness for those suffering from hormone imbalance: www.bodylogicmd.com. You might also consider finding a functional medical practitioner.

Naturopathy

Naturopathy is based on the belief that the body is innately capable of recovering from injury and disease, since health is its natural state. Most naturopaths incorporate elements from various alternative methods, including homeopathy, herbal medicines, acupuncture, nutrition therapy, and bodywork. Naturopathy has its roots in ancient medicinal practices, but took form as a separate discipline in Germany in the 19th century. Founded on the precepts of a medical regimen of hydrotherapy, exercise, fresh air, sunlight, and herbal remedies, this system has evolved today to include a wide spectrum of holistic practitioners. Here are two resources to find one in your area:

- American Association of Naturopathic Physicians (www.naturopathic.org)

- Bastyr University Naturopathic Medicine Graduate Program (www.bastyr.edu)

SUPPLEMENTS

Look for pharmaceutical-grade supplements. Companies such as the following make high-quality products, many of which I recommend to my patients.

- Biotics Research (www.bioticsresearch.com)

- Designs for Health (www.designsforhealth.com)

- Douglas Laboratories (www.douglaslabs.com)

- Emerson Ecologics—Ther-biotic (www.emersonecologics.com)

- Integrative Therapeutics (www.integrativeinc.com)

- J.R. Carlson Laboratories (www.carlsonlabs.com)

- Life Extension Foundation (www.lef.org)

- Metagenics (www.metagenics.com)

- Nutrition Dynamics (www.nutritiondynamics.com)

- Ortho Molecular Products (www.orthomolecularproducts.com)

- Pure Encapsulations (www.bayho.com/c/pure-encapsulations.html)

- Scientific Botanicals (www.scientificbotanicals.net)

- Standard Process (www.standardprocess.com)

- Thorne Research (www.thorne.com)

- Women to Women (www.womentowomen.com)

- XYMOGEN (www.xymogen.com)

WEBSITES

Meditation

- www.chopra.com/meditation

- www.freemeditations.com

- www.meditationoasis.com

Music

- www.hayhouse.com

- www.healingsounds.com

- www.soundfeelings.com

Self-Help Publications and Audio Products

- www.hayhouse.com

Visualization

- www.hayhouse.com

- www.visualization-techniques.com

- www.crystalsbay.net

Additional Information

- www.thework.com (Byron Katie)
- www.hoffmaninstitute.org (Hoffman Process)
- www.MarcellePick.com
- www.pbs.org
- www.plotinus.com
- www.womentowomen.com

Sexuality

- Mama Gena's School of Womanly Arts (www.mamagenas.com)
- www.bermanandberman.com
- www.goodvibes.com
- www.passionparties.com
- Victoria's Secret—great lingerie (www.victoriassecret.com)
- www.understandmen.com (Alison Armstrong—PAX programs)
- Ballroom dancing: www.ballroomdancers.com; http://ballroomdancers.info; www.learnandmaster.com/ballroom-dance; www.ballroomdance101.com
- Pelvic PT resource: (www.functionabilitypt.com/womens_pelvic_floor_dysfunction.htm)
- Tantric breathing with Barbara Carrellas (http://urbantantra.org)
- Tantric breathing (www.newfrontier.com/nepal/pranayama.htm)
- Edible massage oils (www.lovepotions.com)

BOOKS

- Colucci, Anna F. *PMS Self Help: A Self-Help Book To Help You Deal With Your Premenstrual Symptoms With A Guide To Several Medication Cures For PMS And Natural Remedies . . . Help You Get Fast And Lasting Relief For PMS* (Lexington, KY: Anna F. Colucci, May 17, 2012).

- Dell, Diana L., M.D., F.A.C.O.G., and Carol Svec. *The PMDD Phenomenon: Breakthrough Treatments for Premenstrual Dysphoric Disorder (PMDD) and Extreme Premenstrual Syndrome* (New York: Contemporary Books, 2002).

- Hahn, Linaya. *PMS—Solving the Puzzle: Sixteen Causes of Premenstrual Syndrome and What to Do About It* (Evanston, IL: Chicago Spectrum Press, 1995).

- Hoffman, Bob. *No One Is to Blame: Freedom from Compulsive Self-Defeating Behavior; the Discoveries of the Quadrinity Process* (Oakland, CA: Recycling Books, 1988).

- Hyman, Mark, M.D. *The Blood Sugar Solution: The UltraHealthy Program for Losing Weight, Preventing Disease, and Feeling Great Now!* (New York: Little, Brown, 2012).

- James, E. L. *Fifty Shades of Grey: Book One of the Fifty Shades Trilogy* (New York: Vintage Books, 2011).

- Joannides, Paul, Psy.D., and Gröss Daerick Sr. *Guide to Getting It On! A Book About the Wonders of Sex* (Waldport, OR: Goofy Foot Press, 2011).

- Landa, Jennifer, M.D. *The Sex Drive Solution for Women: Dr. Jen's Power Plan to Fire Up Your Libido* (Ocala, FL: Atlantic Publishing Group, 2012).

- McClellan, Stephanie, M.D., and Beth Hamilton, M.D. with Diane Reverand. *The Ultimate Stress-Relief Plan for Women* (New York: Free Press, 2010).

- Northrup, Christiane, M.D. *The Secret Pleasures of Menopause* (Carlsbad, CA: Hay House, 2008).

- ———. *The Wisdom of Menopause: Creating Physical and Emotional Health During the Change* (New York: Bantam, 2012).

- ———. *Women's Bodies, Women's Wisdom* (New York: Bantam, 2010).

- Randolf, C. W., Jr., M.D., and Genie James, M.M.Sc. *From Belly Fat to Belly Flat* (Deerfield Beach, FL: Health Communications, 2008).

- ———. *From Hormone Hell to Hormone Well* (Deerfield Beach, FL: Health Communications, 2009).

- Redmond, Geoffrey, M.D. *It's Your Hormones* (New York: HarperCollins, 2005).

- ———. *The Good News About Women's Hormones* (New York: Warner Books, 1995).

- Reiss, Uzzi, M.D., OB/GYN, with Martin Zucker. *Natural Hormone Balance for Women* (New York: Pocket Books, 2001).

- Schnarch, Dr. David. *Intimacy & Desire: Awaken the Passion in Your Relationship* (New York: Sterling Productions, 2009).

- Schwarzbein, Diana, M.D., and Nancy Deville. *The Schwarzbein Principle: The Truth About Losing Weight, Being Healthy, and Feeling Younger* (Deerfield Beach, FL: Health Communications, 1999).

- Selye, Hans, M.D. *The Stress of Life* (New York: McGraw-Hill, 1984).

- Smith, Pamela, M.D., M.P.H. *What You Must Know About Women's Hormones* (Garden City Park, NY: Square One Publishers, 2010).

- Stanton, Alicia, M.D., and Vera Tweed. *Hormone Harmony* (Los Angeles, CA: Healthy Life Library, 2009).

- Stanton, Alicia, M.D. *The Complete Idiot's Guide to Hormone Weight Loss* (New York: Alpha Penguin, 2011).

- Taylor, Diana, R.N., Ph.D., and Stacey Colino. *Taking Back the Month: A Personalized Solution for Managing PMS and Enhancing Your Health* (New York: Berkley, 2002).

- Welch, Dr. Claudia, M.S.O.M. *Balance Your Hormones, Balance Your Life* (Cambridge, MA: Da Capo Press, 2011).

CONVERSION CHARTS

Standard Cup	Fine Powder (e.g., flour)	Grain (e.g., rice)	Granular (e.g., sugar)	Liquid Solids (e.g., butter)	Liquid (e.g., milk)
1	140 g	150 g	190 g	200 g	240 ml
¾	105 g	113 g	143 g	150 g	180 ml
⅔	93 g	100 g	125 g	133 g	160 ml
½	70 g	75 g	95 g	100 g	120 ml
⅓	47 g	50 g	63 g	67 g	80 ml
¼	35 g	38 g	48 g	50 g	60 ml
⅛	18 g	19 g	24 g	25 g	30 ml

Useful Equivalents for Liquid Ingredients by Volume					
¼ tsp				1 ml	
½ tsp				2 ml	
1 tsp				5 ml	
3 tsp	1 tbsp		½ fl oz	15 ml	
	2 tbsp	⅛ cup	1 fl oz	30 ml	
	4 tbsp	¼ cup	2 fl oz	60 ml	
	5⅓ tbsp	⅓ cup	3 fl oz	80 ml	
	8 tbsp	½ cup	4 fl oz	120 ml	
	10⅔ tbsp	⅔ cup	5 fl oz	160 ml	
	12 tbsp	¾ cup	6 fl oz	180 ml	
	16 tbsp	1 cup	8 fl oz	240 ml	
	1 pt	2 cups	16 fl oz	480 ml	
	1 qt	4 cups	32 fl oz	960 ml	
			33 fl oz	1000 ml	1 l

Useful Equivalents for Dry Ingredients by Weight

To convert ounces to grams, multiply the number of ounces by 30.

1 oz	1/16 lb	30 g
4 oz	1/4 lb	120 g
8 oz	1/2 lb	240 g
12 oz	3/4 lb	360 g
16 oz	1 lb	480 g

Useful Equivalents for Cooking/Oven Temperatures

Process	Fahrenheit	Celsius	Gas Mark
Freeze Water	32° F	0° C	
Room Temperature	68° F	20° C	
Boil Water	212° F	100° C	
Bake	325° F	160° C	3
	350° F	180° C	4
	375° F	190° C	5
	400° F	200° C	6
	425° F	220° C	7
	450° F	230° C	8
Broil			Grill

Useful Equivalents for Length

To convert inches to centimeters, multiply the number of inches by 2.5.

1 in			2.5 cm	
6 in	1/2 ft		15 cm	
12 in	1 ft		30 cm	
36 in	3 ft	1 yd	90 cm	
40 in			100 cm	1 m

BIBLIOGRAPHY

CHAPTER 1

Andersson, M., B. de Benoist, L. Rogers. "Epidemiology of iodine deficiency: Salt iodisation and iodine status." *Best Pract Res Clin Endocrinol Metab,* February 2010; 24(1): 1–11.

Aubertin-Leheudre, M., S. Gorbach, M. Woods et al. "Fat/Fiber intakes and sex hormones in healthy premenopausal women in USA." *J Steroid Biochem Mol Biol,* November 2008; 112(1–3): 32–39.

Bulun, S. E., K. Zeitoun, K. Takayama et al. "Estrogen production in endometriosis and use of aromatase inhibitors to treat endometriosis." *Endoc Relat Cancer,* June 1999; 6(2): 293–301.

Chiu, K. C., A. Chu, V. L. Go et al. "Hypovitaminosis D is associated with insulin resistance and beta cell dysfunction." *Am J Clin Nutr,* May 2004; 79(5): 820–5.

Dante, G., F. Facchinetti. "Herbal treatments for alleviating premenstrual symptoms: a systematic review." *J Psychosom Obstet Gynaecol,* March 2011; 32(1): 42–51.

Freeman, E. W. "Therapeutic management of premenstrual syndrome." *Expert Opin Pharmacother,* December 2010; 11(17): 2879–89.

Geller, S. E., L. P. Shulman, R. B. van Breemen et al. "Safety and Efficacy of Black Cohosh and Red Clover for the Management of Vasomotor Symptoms: A Randomized Controlled Trial." *Menopause,* 2009; 16(6): 1156–66.

Greenlee, H., C. Atkinson, F. Z. Stanczyk et al. "A pilot and feasibility study on the effects of naturopathic botanical and dietary interventions on sex steroid hormone metabolism in premenopausal women." *Cancer Epidemiol Biomarkers Prev,* August 2007; 16(8): 1601–09.

Jacobson, J. S., A. B. Troxel, J. Evans et al. "Randomized trial of black cohosh for the treatment of hot flashes among women with a history of breast cancer." *J Clin Oncol,* May 15, 2001; 19(10): 2739–45.

Ma, L., S. Lin, R. Chen, X. Wang. "Treatment of moderate to severe premenstrual syndrome with Vitex agnus castus (BNO 1095) in Chinese women." *Gynecol Endocrinol,* August 2010; 26(8): 612–16.

Miyai, K., T. Tokushige, M. Kondo; Iodine Research Group. "Suppression of thyroid function during ingestion of seaweed 'Kombu' (Laminaria japonoca) in normal Japanese adults." *Endocr J,* December 2008; 55(6): 1103–8.

Parazzini, F., F. Chiaffarino, M. Surace et al. "Selected food intake and risk of endometriosis." *Hum Reprod,* 2004; 19 (8): 1755–59.

Rose, D. P., M. Lubin, J. M. Connolly. "Effects of diet supplementation with wheat bran on serum estrogen levels in the follicular and luteal phases of the menstrual cycle." *Nutrition,* June 1997; 13(6): 535–39.

Teas, J., L. E. Braverman, M. S. Kurzer et al. "Seaweed and soy: companion foods in Asian cuisine and their effects on thyroid function in American women." *J Med Food,* March 2007; 10(1): 90–100.

Toth, B. "Stress, inflammation and endometriosis: are patients stuck between a rock and a hard place?" *J Mol Med,* 2010(88): 223–25.

Utian, W. H. "A decade post WHI, menopausal hormone therapy comes full circle—need for independent commission." *Climacteric,* August 2012; 15(4): 320–25.

Vines, A., T. A. Myduc, D. A. Esserman. "The Association between Self-Reported Major Life Events and the Presence of Uterine Fibroids." *Womens Health Issues,* July–August 2010; 20(4): 294–98.

Waddell, B. J., P. C. O'Leary. "Distribution and metabolism of topically applied progesterone in a rat model." *J Steroid Biochem Mol Biol,* April 2002; 80(4–5): 449–55.

Worthman, C., J. Stallings, L. Hofman. "Sensitive Salivary Estradiol Assay for Monitoring Ovarian Function." *Clin Chem,* 1990(36/10): 1769–73.

CHAPTER 2

Bennett, J., A. Pope. *The Pill: Are You Sure It's for You?* (Crows Nest, NSW, Australia: Allen & Unwin, 2008).

Bruning, P. F., J. M. Bonfrèr, P. A. van Noord et al. "Insulin resistance and breast-cancer risk." *Int J Cancer,* October, 21, 1992; 52(4): 511–16.

Bulun, S. E., K. Zeitoun, K. Takayama et al. "Estrogen production in endometriosis and use of aromatase inhibitors to treat endometriosis." *Endoc Relat Cancer,* June 1999; 6(2): 293–301.

Davidson, N. E. "Environmental Estrogens and Breast Cancer Risk." *Curr Opin Oncol,* September 1998; 10(5): 475–78.

Davis, D. L., H. L. Bradlow. "Can Environmental Estrogens Cause Breast Cancer?" *Scientific American,* October 1995; 273(4): 167–72.

Gozansky, W. S., J. S. Lynn, M. L. Laudenslager et al. "Salivary cortisol determined by enzyme immunoassay is preferable to serum total cortisol for assessment of dynamic hypothalamic-pituitary-adrenal axis activity." *Clin Endocrinol (Oxf),* September 2005; 63(3): 336–41.

Greenlee, H., C. Atkinson, F. Z. Stanczyk et al. "A pilot and feasibility study on the effects of naturopathic botanical and dietary interventions on sex steroid hormone metabolism in premenopausal women." *Cancer Epidemiol Biomarkers Prev,* August 2007; 16(8): 1601–09.

Gröschl, M. "Current status of salivary hormone analysis." *Clin Chem,* November 2008; 54(11): 1759–69.

Lee, E., S. Oh, M. Kim et al. "Modulatory effects of alpha- and gamma-tocopherols on 4-hydroxyestradiol induced oxidative stresses in MCF-10A breast epithelial cells." *Nutr Res Pract*, Fall 2009; 3(3): 185–91.

Low Dog, T., D. Riley, T. Carter. "An integrative approach to menopause." *Altern Ther Health Med*, July–August 2001; 7(4): 45–57.

Miller, G. E., S. Cohen, A. K. Ritchey. "Chronic psychological stress and the regulation of pro-inflammatory cytokines: a glucocorticoid-resistance model." *Health Psychol*, November 2002; 21(6): 531–41.

O'Leary, P., P. Feddema, K. Chan et al. "Salivary, but not serum or urinary levels of progesterone are elevated after topical application of progesterone cream to pre- and postmenopausal women." *Clin Endocrinol (Oxf)*, November 2000; 53(5): 615–20.

Sowers, M. R., S. Crawford, D. S. McConnell et al. "Selected diet and lifestyle factors are associated with estrogen metabolites in a multiracial/ethnic population of women." *J Nutr*, June 2006; 136(6): 1588–95.

CHAPTER 3

Bulun, S. E., Z. Fang, G. Imir et al. "Aromatase and endometriosis." *Semin Reprod Med*, February 2004; 22(1): 45–50.

Gozansky, W. S., J. S. Lynn, M. L. Laudenslager et al. "Salivary cortisol determined by enzyme immunoassay is preferable to serum total cortisol for assessment of dynamic hypothalamic-pituitary-adrenal axis activity." *Clin Endocrinol (Oxf)*, September 2005; 63(3): 336–41.

Miller, G. E., S. Cohen, A. K. Ritchey. "Chronic psychological stress and the regulation of pro-inflammatory cytokines: a glucocorticoid-resistance model." *Health Psychol*, November 2002; 21(6): 531–41.

Riad-Fahmy, D., G. F. Read, R. F. Walker. "Salivary steroid assays for assessing variation in endocrine activity." *J Steroid Biochem*, July 1983; 19(1A): 265–72.

Sowers, M. R., S. Crawford, D. S. McConnell et al. "Selected diet and lifestyle factors are associated with estrogen metabolites in a multiracial/ethnic population of women." *J Nutr*, June 2006; 136(6): 1588–95.

CHAPTER 4

Atmaca, M., S. Kumru, E. Tezcan. "Fluoxetine versus Vitex agnus castus extract in the treatment of premenstrual dysphoric disorder." *Hum Psychopharmacol*, April 2003; 18(3): 191–95.

Aubertin-Leheudre, M., S. Gorbach, M. Woods et al. "Fat/Fiber intakes and sex hormones in healthy premenopausal women in USA." *J Steroid Biochem Mol Biol*, November 2008; 112(1–3): 32–39.

Begley, Sharon. "The Estrogen Complex." *Newsweek,* March 21, 1994: 77.

Beral, V., Million Women Study Collaborators. "Breast Cancer and Hormone-replacement Therapy in the Million Women Study." *Lancet,* August 9, 2003; 362(9382): 419–27.

Bernard, N. D., A. R. Scialli, D. Hurlock et al. "Diet and sex-hormone binding globulin, dysmenorrheal and premenstrual symptoms." *Obstet Gynecol,* February 2000; 95(2): 245–50.

Bolaji, I. I, D. F. Tallon, E . O'Dwyer, et al. "Assessment of bioavailability of oral micronized progesterone using a salivary progesterone enzymeimmunoassay." *Gynecol Endocrinol.* June 1993; 7(2): 101–10.

Burry, K. A., P. E. Patton, K. Hermsmeyer. "Percutaneous absorption of progesterone in postmenopausal women treated with transdermal estrogen." *Am J Obstet Gynecol,* June 1999; 180(6Pt 1): 1504–11.

Chiu, K. C., A. Chu, V. L. Go, et al. "Hypovitaminosis D is associated with insulin resistance and beta cell dysfunction." *Am J Clin Nutr,* May 2004; 79(5): 820–25.

Dante, G., F. Facchinetti. "Herbal treatments for alleviating premenstrual symptoms: a systematic review." *J Pysychosom Obstet Gynaecol,* March 2011; 32(1): 42–51.

Davidson, N. E. "Environmental Estrogens and Breast Cancer Risk." *Curr Opin Oncol,* September 1998; 10(5): 475–78.

Fowke, J. H., C. Longcope, J. R. Hebert. "Brassica vegetable consumption shifts estrogen metabolism in healthy postmenopausal women." *Cancer Epidemiol Biomarkers Prev,* August 2000; 9(8): 773–79.

Greenlee, H., C. Atkinson, F. Z. Stanczyk et al. "A pilot and feasibility study on the effects of naturopathic botanical and dietary interventions on sex steroid hormone metabolism in premenopausal women." *Cancer Epidemiol Biomarkers Prev,* August 2007; 16(8): 1601–09.

Jacobson, J. S., A. B. Troxel, J. Evans et al. "Randomized trial of black cohosh for the treatment of hot flashes among women with a history of breast cancer." *J Clin Oncol,* May 15, 2001; 19(10): 2739–45.

Kolata, Gina with Melody Petersen. "Hormone Replacement Study A Shock to the Medical System." *New York Times,* July 10, 2002.

Lappano, R., C. Rosano, P. De Marco et al. "Estriol acts as a GPR30 antagonist in estrogen receptor-negative breast cancer cells." *Mol Cell Endocrinol,* May 14, 2010; 320(1–2): 162–70.

Li, Y., T. Zhang, H. Korkaya et al. "Sulforaphane, a dietary component of broccoli/broccoli sprouts, inhibits breast cancer stem cells." *Clin Cancer Res,* May 1, 2010; 16(9): 2580–90.

Ma, L., S. Lin, R. Chen et al. "Treatment of moderate to severe premenstrual syndrome with Vitex agnus castus (BNO 1095) in Chinese women." *Gynecol Endocrinol,* August 2010; 26(8): 612–16.

Majumdar, S. R., E. A. Almasi, R. S. Stafford. "Promotion and prescribing of hormone therapy after report of harm by the Women's Health Initiative." *J Am Med Assoc,* October 27, 2004; 292(16): 1983–88.

Miyai, K., T. Tokushige, M. Kondo; Iodine Research Group. "Suppression of thyroid function during ingestion of seaweed 'Kombu' (Laminaria japonoca) in normal Japanese adults." *Endocrine Journal*, December 2008; 55(6): 1103–8.

Obi, N., J. Chang-Claude, J. Berger et al. "The Use of Herbal Preparations to Alleviate Climacteric Disorders and Risk of Postmenopausal Breast Cancer in a German Case-Control Study." *Cancer Epidemiol Biomarkers Prev*, 2009; 18: 2207–13.

O'Leary, P., P. Feddema, K. Chan et al. "Salivary, but not serum or urinary levels of progesterone are elevated after topical application of progesterone cream to pre- and postmenopausal women." *Clin Endocrinol (Oxf)*, November 2000; 53(5): 615–20.

Remer, T., A. Neubert, F. Manz. "Increased risk of iodine deficiency with vegetarian nutrition." *Br J Nutr*, January 1999; 81(1): 45–49.

Robb, E. L., J. A. Stuart. "Resveratrol interacts with estrogen receptor-ß to inhibit cell replicative growth and enhance stress resistance by upregulating mitochondrial superoxide dismutase." *Free Radic Biol Med*, April 2011; 50(7): 821–31.

Rose, D. P., M. Lubin, J. M. Connolly. "Effects of diet supplementation with wheat bran on serum estrogen levels in the follicular and luteal phases of the menstrual cycle." *Nutrition*, June 1997; 13(6): 535–9.

Stoddard, F. R., II, A. D. Brooks, B. A. Eskin et al. "Iodine Alters Gene Expression in the MCF7 Breast Cancer Cell Line: Evidence for an Anti-Estrogen Effect of Iodine." *Int J Med Sci*, 2008; 5(4): 189–96.

Sturgeon, S. R., J. L. Heersink, S. L. Volpe et al. "Effect of dietary flaxseed on serum levels of estrogens and androgens in postmenopausal women." *Nutr Cancer*, 2008; 60(5): 612–18.

Utian, W. H. "A decade post WHI, menopausal hormone therapy comes full circle—need for independent commission." *Climacteric*, August 2012; 15(4): 320–25.

Waddell, B. J., P. C. O'Leary. "Distribution and metabolism of topically applied progesterone in a rat model." *J Steroid Biochem Mol Biol*, April 2002; 80(4–5): 449–55.

Wang, Y., K. W. Lee, F. L. Chan et al. "The red wine polyphenol resveratrol displays bilevel inhibition on aromatase in breast cancer cells." *Toxicol Sci*, July 2006; 92(1): 71–77.

Wuttke, W., H. Jarry, V. Christoffel et al. "Chaste tree pharmacology and clinical indications." *Phytomedicine*, May 2003; 10(4): 348–57.

CHAPTER 5

Bruning, P. F., J. M. Bonfrèr, P. A. van Noord et al. "Insulin resistance and breast-cancer risk." *Int J Cancer*, October 21, 1992; 52(4): 511–16.

Bulun, S. E., K. Zeitoun, K. Takayama et al. "Estrogen production in endometriosis and use of aromatase inhibitors to treat endometriosis." *Endoc Relat Cancer*, June 1999; 6(2): 293–301.

Chakraborti, C. K. "Vitamin D as a promising anticancer agent." *Indian J Pharmacol,* April 2011; 43(2): 113–20.

Cho, E., W. Y. Chen, D. J. Hunter et al. "Red Meat Intake and Risk of Breast Cancer Among Premenopausal Women." *Arch Intern Med,* 2006; 166: 2253–59.

Foster, W.G. "Endocrine toxicants including 2,3,7,8-terachlorodibenzo-p-dioxin (TCDD) and dioxin-like chemicals and endometriosis: is there a link?" *J Toxicol Environ Health B Crit Rev,* March 2008; 11(3–4): 177–87.

Geller, S. E., L. P. Shulman, R. B. van Breemen et al. "Safety and Efficacy of Black Cohosh and Red Clover for the Management of Vasomotor Symptoms: A Randomized Controlled Trial."*Menopause,* 2009; 16(6): 1156–66.

Jacobson, J. S., A. B. Troxel, J. Evans et al. "Randomized trial of black cohosh for the treatment of hot flashes among women with a history of breast cancer." *J Clin Oncol,* May 15, 2001; 19(10): 2739–45.

Kaaks, R. "Nutrition, hormones, and breast cancer: is insulin the missing link?" *Cancer Causes Control*, November 1996; 7(6): 605–25.

Lawlor, D. A., G. D. Smith, S. Ebrahim. "Hyperinsulinaemia and increased risk of breast cancer: findings from the British Women's Heart and Health Study." *Cancer Causes Control,* April 2004; 15(3): 267–75.

Obi, N., J. Chang-Claude, J. Berger et al. "The Use of Herbal Preparations to Alleviate Climacteric Disorders and Risk of Postmenopausal Breast Cancer in a German Case-Control Study." *Cancer Epidemiol Biomarkers Prev,* 2009; 18: 2207–13.

The Endogenous Hormones and Breast Cancer Collaborative Group. "Endogenous sex hormones and breast cancer in postmenopausal women: reanalysis of nine prospective studies." *J Natl Cancer Inst,* April 17, 2002; 94 (8): 606–16.

Thier, R, T. Brüning, P. H. Roos et al. "Markers of genetic susceptibility in human environmental hygiene and toxicology: the role of selected CYP, NAT and GST genes." *Int J Hyg Environ Health,* June 2003; 206(3): 149–71.

Utian, W. H. "A decade post WHI, menopausal hormone therapy comes full circle—need for independent commission." *Climacteric,* 2012; 15: 320–25.

> This article is a reconsideration of the 2001 Women's Health Initiative study. When the study was reconsidered, many conventional practitioners were extremely angry. They claimed that because of the flawed interpretation of this study, thousands of women had avoided HRT—treatments that potentially might have prevented heart disease and bone loss among these women. The critique of the study seemed to validate the position of those practitioners who had supported HRT all along.
>
> I agree that the study was seriously misinterpreted. Its claims about the dangers of HRT seemed to be significantly overstated and based on a flawed interpretation of the data. Some practitioners concluded that HRT was safe and went on to prescribe it for their patients. I personally prefer to prescribe hormones that mimic as closely as possible the hormones in the human body, so while I also prescribe hormones for my patients, I have chosen to rely on bioidentical rather than conventional versions of those hormones.

Venugopal, D., M. Zahid, P. C. Mailander et al. "Reduction of estrogen-induced transformation of mouse mammary epithelial cells by N-acetylcysteine." *J Steroid Biochem Mol Biol,* March 2008; 109(1–2): 22–30.

Zeyneloglu, H. B., A. Arici, D. L. Olive. "Environmental toxins and endometriosis." *Obstet Gynecol Clin North Am,* June 1997; 24(2): 307–29.

CHAPTER 6

Halldorsson, T. I., D. Rytter, L. S. Haug et al. "Prenatal exposure to perfluorooctanoate and risk of overweight at 20 years of age: a prospective cohort study." *Environ Health Perspect,* May 2012; 120(5): 668–73.

Hayes, T. B., V. Khoury, A. Narayan et al. "Atrazine induces complete feminization and chemical castration in male African clawed frogs (Xenopus laevis)." *Proc Natl Acad Sci USA,* March 9, 2010; 107(10): 4612–17.

Hayes, T. B., A. Collins, M. Lee et al. "Hermaphroditic, demasculinized frogs after exposure to the herbicide atrazine at low ecologically relevant doses." *Proc Natl Acad Sci USA,* April 16, 2002; 99(8): 5476–80.

Lang, I. A., T. S. Galloway, A. Scarlett et al. "Association of urinary bisphenol A concentration with medical disorders and laboratory abnormalities in adults." *J Am Med Assoc,* September 12, 2008; 300(11): 1303–10.

Lee, D., I. Lee, K. Song et al. "Association between serum concentrations of persistent organic pollutants and insulin resistance among nondiabetic adults." *Diabetes Care* 2007; 30: 622–28.

Lim, J. S., D. H. Lee, J. Y. Park et al. "A strong interaction between serum GGT and obesity on the risk of prevalent type 2 diabetes: results from the Third National Health and Nutrition Examination Survey." *Clin Chem,* 2007; 53(6): 1092–98.

Lim, S. S. Y. Ahn, I. C. Song et al. "Chronic Exposure to the herbicide, Atrazine, causes mitochondrial dysfunction and insulin resistance." *PloS ONE,* April 2009; 4(4): e5186.

Lim, S., Y. M. Cho, K. S. Park et al. "Persistent organic pollutants, mitochondrial dysfunction, and metabolic syndrome. Mitochondrial Research in Translational Medicine." *Ann NY Acad Sci,* 2010 (1201): 166–76.

Meliker, J. R., R. L. Wahl, L. L. Cameron et al. "Arsenic in drinking water and cerebrovascular disease, diabetes mellitus, and kidney disease in Michigan: a standardized mortality ratio analysis." *Environ Health,* February 2, 2007; 6: 4.

Ruzzin, J., R. Petersen, E. Meugnier et al. "Persistent organic pollutant exposure leads to insulin resistance syndrome." *Environ Health Perspect,* April 2010; 118(4): 465–71.

Vom Saal, F. S., J. P. Myers. "Bisphenol, A and risk of metabolic disorders." *J Am Med Assoc,* September 17, 2008; 300(11): 1353–54.

INDEX

INDEX OF RECIPES

ACKNOWLEDGMENTS

Writing this book was a journey, not without its struggles, but it was always inspired by my deep yearning to change the world of women's health, and by my deepest desire to help women understand that they have much more power to change their health than they realize. They can, in fact, expect to be well into old age.

I am indebted to my extraordinary team at Hay House, who has always believed in me, especially Reid Tracy, who continues to encourage me to reach for the sky, and Louise Hay, who is a mentor for all of us. Hay House: Hats off to all of you. You are amazing!

My amazing editorial team, Patty Gift with whom I always love working, Peter Guzzardi for cleaning up the edits and being willing to take a risk. To the wonderful Rachel Kranz for your tireless efforts to get the words just right. How you keep the hours you do I will never know! To Janis Vallely, who so often knows how to take the right approach. And thank you, Stephanie Tade, who always acts on my behalf and knows how to put the package together. My publicists, Beth Grossman and Jason Beyers, for your wonderful words of gentle advice.

Thank you so much for those that have inspired me and helped me get clearer that getting the word out is essential, Dr. Jeff Bland, who asks more of all of us in a scientific way. Dr. Mark Hyman for having the courage to pave the way. To Brendon Burchard and the Inner Circle for encouraging me to go for it. Own it. Dr. Frank Lipman, Dr. Liz Lipski, Dr. Patrick Hanaway, Dr. Dixie Mills, Dr. Oz, and Oprah Winfrey, whose words continue to inspire me to go beyond and take risks.

To Michael Allosso, for holding the mirror and holding me accountable. To Aita Passmore, for telling me the truth. To JJ Virgin, for holding the torch and making the amazing connections. You are an inspiration. All those at IFM: teachers and practitioners alike that urge us to be impeccable, to take the word out and create a world of wellness rather than dis-ease.

To my inner circle of support, without you I could not have done this. Julie Cunningham, thanks for always being there and standing strong by my side. Sally McCue, for reminding me about my truth and how important it is to pursue our dreams. Jennie, for keeping me honest and on the right path. My Monday night group, for always helping to put things in perspective.

To all my friends, who continue to support me in so many ways. Nalini Chilkov, who always holds the light and has become the sister I never had. Suzanne Bennett, who continues to encourage me to go beyond. Alan Christianson, whose wonderful laugh and support remind me to have fun too.

To Concordia: Jeff, Richard, and the team for always wanting to get the message out in cyberspace and for doing it so well

To Raz, Liza, and the Hoffman Institute, for showing me the way and for continuing to support healing in the world.

To my wonderful dance group: Wayne, Carolyn, Cathy, Donna, Irene, Dana, Charlie, and Rob, who keep my happiness meter up. Rene Noel, for taking me under his wing and asking me to be better, and allowing me to laugh at my mistakes.

A special thank you to my staff at Women to Women. I know at times it was difficult when the book push was on: Carrie, Cate, Holly, Rachel, Susan, Laura, Sue, Jodie, Rafina, Brenda, Karen, Christy, Jane, Kay, and Shelley.

And to Donna Poulin, without whom much of this would not have been possible. Her ingenious ability to create recipes is something I am in awe of, and her amazing friendship is the greatest gift.

To Dr. Joe Lamb, who helped with the initial edits so I felt secure in the scientific data, without his endless support, the book would have been much harder. Thank you also for always having my back; your friendship and support made the difference.

And lastly to my wonderful children and family who inspire me to make things different for the generations to follow. Katya, for being the amazing, sensitive woman that you are, the daughter that urged me to go further. Micah, for being oh so creative and for being willing to share your gifts and support to the world. And Josh for holding the light, pushing the envelope, and striving to be the healer that you are. Ralph, for always being there; Evan, for reminding me what is possible; Rene, for being such a supportive sister-in-law, and my dad for giving me the strength to ask the hard questions and demanding personal and professional excellence.

I am oh so grateful to all who have been and continue to be in my path. I am truly blessed.

ABOUT THE AUTHOR

Marcelle Pick, OB/GYN and pediatric NP, grew up in Australia, surrounded by aboriginal cave drawings, healthy home-cooked meals, sunshine, and beautiful crystal water. It was there that she gained an appreciation for the healing power of nature, whole foods, and positive thinking.

After earning a B.S. in Nursing from the University of New Hampshire, a B.A. in Psychology from the University of New Hampshire, and her M.S. in Nursing from Boston College–Harvard Medical School, Marcelle co-founded the world-renowned Women to Women Clinic in Yarmouth, Maine, with a vision to change the way in which women's health care is delivered. In her practice, Marcelle undertakes an integrative approach that not only treats illness but also helps women make choices to prevent disease. She has successfully worked with thousands of women to help them create wellness in their lives.

In 2001, Marcelle co-founded Women to Women's Personal Program, exclusively available at www.womentowomen.com. This site is dedicated to helping women navigate their most common health concerns. This multimedia collection gives women well-researched information so that they are able to make informed decisions about their health—and, in some instances, transform their lives.

Marcelle is a prolific writer and passionate advocate for women's health. She is a regular contributor to womentowomen.com and *The Huffington Post,* and she makes frequent media appearances, including *The Dr. OZ Show* and Martha Stewart's *Whole Living,* to encourage women to take control of their diet and lifestyle.

Is It Me or My Hormones? is Marcelle's third book. Her two previous best-selling books, *The Core Balance Diet* and *Is It Me or My Adrenals?* are popular throughout the world. Women everywhere love Marcelle's balanced approach to health care. Her writing and her work focus on the importance of a healthy diet and lifestyle and looking at the impact of emotions on physical health.

Marcelle currently lives in southern Maine, enjoying time with her children, boating on the beautiful ocean, and her newfound love of ballroom dance.

Website: **www.womentowomen.com**

Hay House Titles of Related Interest

YOU CAN HEAL YOUR LIFE, the movie, starring Louise L. Hay & Friends
(available as a 1-DVD program and an expanded 2-DVD set)
Watch the trailer at: **www.LouiseHayMovie.com**

THE SHIFT, the movie,
starring Dr. Wayne W. Dyer
(available as a 1-DVD program and an expanded 2-DVD set)
Watch the trailer at: **www.DyerMovie.com**

■ ■

ALL IS WELL: Heal Your Body with Medicine, Affirmations, and Intuition,
by Louise L. Hay and Mona Lisa Schulz, M.D., Ph.D.

INNER PEACE FOR BUSY WOMEN: Balancing Work, Family, and Your Inner Life,
by Joan Z. Borysenko, Ph.D.

INTEGRATIVE WELLNESS RULES: A Simple Guide to Healthy Living, by Dr. Jim Nicolai

THE SECRET PLEASURES OF MENOPAUSE, by Christiane Northrup, M.D.

All of the above are available at your local bookstore,
or may be ordered by contacting Hay House (see next page).

■ ■

We hope you enjoyed this Hay House book. If you'd like
to receive our online catalog featuring additional information on
Hay House books and products, or if you'd like to find out more
about the Hay Foundation, please contact:

Hay House, Inc., P.O. Box 5100, Carlsbad, CA 92018-5100
(760) 431-7695 or (800) 654-5126
(760) 431-6948 (fax) or (800) 650-5115 (fax)
www.hayhouse.com® • **www.hayfoundation.org**

■ ■

Published and distributed in Australia by: Hay House Australia Pty. Ltd., 18/36 Ralph St.,
Alexandria NSW 2015 • *Phone:* 612-9669-4299 • *Fax:* 612-9669-4144 • www.hayhouse.com.au

Published and distributed in the United Kingdom by: Hay House UK, Ltd., 292B Kensal Rd.,
London W10 5BE • *Phone:* 44-20-8962-1230 • *Fax:* 44-20-8962-1239 • www.hayhouse.co.uk

Published and distributed in the Republic of South Africa by: Hay House SA (Pty), Ltd., P.O. Box 990,
Witkoppen 2068 • *Phone/Fax:* 27-11-467-8904 • www.hayhouse.co.za

Published in India by: Hay House Publishers India, Muskaan Complex, Plot No. 3, B-2, Vasant Kunj,
New Delhi 110 070 • *Phone:* 91-11-4176-1620 • *Fax:* 91-11-4176-1630 • www.hayhouse.co.in

Distributed in Canada by: Raincoast, 9050 Shaughnessy St., Vancouver, B.C. V6P 6E5
Phone: (604) 323-7100 • *Fax:* (604) 323-2600 • www.raincoast.com

■ ■

Take Your Soul on a Vacation

Visit **www.HealYourLife.com®** to regroup, recharge,
and reconnect with your own magnificence.
Featuring blogs, mind-body-spirit news, and life-changing
wisdom from Louise Hay and friends.

Visit **www.HealYourLife.com** today!

Free e-newsletters from Hay House, the Ultimate Resource for Inspiration

Be the first to know about Hay House's dollar deals, free downloads, special offers, affirmation cards, giveaways, contests, and more!

 Get exclusive excerpts from our latest releases and videos from *Hay House Present Moments*.

 Enjoy uplifting personal stories, how-to articles, and healing advice, along with videos and empowering quotes, within *Heal Your Life*.

 Have an inspirational story to tell and a passion for writing? Sharpen your writing skills with insider tips from *Your Writing Life*.

Sign Up Now!

Get inspired, educate yourself, get a complimentary gift, and share the wisdom!

http://www.hayhouse.com/newsletters.php

Visit www.hayhouse.com to sign up today!

 HAY HOUSE

 HAYHOUSE RADIO
radio for your soul

HealYourLife.com ♥